Therese's Dream

I want to thank Doctors Without Borders for providing me with the opportunity to have these remarkable experiences in Africa. Thanks to my family and friends, especially to my sons Arlen and Robert Austin, for encouraging me on these journeys. And my deepest thanks to the people of Africa for sharing their lives with me.

Therese's Dream
Maine to Darfur

A Doctor's Story

Dr. David Austin

Matrika Press
Publisher

ISBN 9781946088109
LIBRARY OF CONGRESS CONTROL NUMBER: 2016915841

MATRIKA PRESS, PUBLISHER

First Edition
Printed in the USA

Contents:

Dave is the most compassionate, caring physician I have known. This is what drew me towards Dave when we met back in Family Medicine residency over 30 years ago. Whether he is working in rural Maine or overseas, helping to serve the poor, Dave does not know from any divide. He sees your uniqueness as a human being and reaches out to make a profound human connection.

To receive one of Dave's emails from overseas means you are going to be taken on an extraordinary adventure into the lives of the native people and their culture. No judgment—just pure acceptance as a friend, with a genuine interest in who you are, where you are from, wanting to meet your family. And when you see him in the clinic, he takes the same regard for you, and he will go to any lengths to see you through your illness or that of your child.

Such a gift that Dave has shared with us—his writing is beautiful and engaging—the world will feel much smaller as Dave helps us touch our universal humanity.

— Alan Weiner, MD

Introduction

Life is precious and fragile. A doctor's primary role, at its best, is to help people regain the delicate balance of health when it has been disrupted by disease, to help maintain and enhance health when present, and to prevent disease when possible. I had the privilege of working as a family doctor in rural Maine from 1989 until 2008. This work was deeply satisfying. My doctoring ranged from prenatal care to hospice care, birth to death, with a focus on the time in-between. I was a relative late comer to medicine. There were no medical people among my known ancestors. My parents were teachers, and I had completed a master's degree in education before a couple of powerful personal experiences — helping to care for my dying stepfather and working as a home health aid for a family friend — turned me toward medical school. From early on I was drawn to the idea of doctoring in parts of the world where people died for lack of care that we take for granted. This idea simmered on my back burner for years, as my two sons grew to adulthood, and was postponed further by the responsibilities of caring for aging parents.

I got a taste of what this work might be like during several two week medical missions to rural areas in the Dominican Republic. A wonderful group of people from the School of Nursing at

the University of Southern Maine (USM) travel
to mountain villages in the Dominican Republic
every six months, providing medical care and health
education to people who lack basic medical resources.
On my first trip in the summer of 2003 I had the great
good fortune of meeting Dave Hotstream, a Peace
Corps volunteer who was serving as a translator for
our group. He was on break from his Peace Corp
project in Restoracion, a small city close to the
Haitian border. He had been helping a Haitian nurse,
Clemencia, who was running a small medical clinic
across the border in Haiti, in the town of Tilori. Dave
was impressed with the medical services that our
group could provide in the Dominican Republic, and
he bemoaned the dearth of supplies available at his
Haitian clinic. I offered to help collect supplies for
the clinic, medications and vitamins, and meet Dave
in six months when the USM group was to return,
and travel to the Haitian clinic to share the wealth.
This was the first of ten trips we made to Clemencia's
clinic in Tilori, returning every six months. We never
spent more than two days at the clinic, but we would
see about 50 of her sicker patients, and leave behind
a good supply of medications. The personal rewards
of these brief medical trips to Haiti were great, and
these experiences helped me believe that, when my
life would allow it, I would be able to commit more
time to this "third world" medical work. We stopped
visiting Tilori after a small hospital was built there.

One story from the Haitian trips demonstrates
the rewards of this work. During one of the two day
trips we cared for an eight month old girl with bad

pneumonia. At the time she qualified as one of the sickest children I had ever seen. We were able to treat her with two days of injectable antibiotics, and leave her with a full course of oral treatment. She was still quite ill when we left. When we returned six months later, Clemencia pointed out a woman with a young toddler and asked if I remembered them. The little girl was vigorous and healthy looking, almost as vibrant as the smile on her mother's face as she showed her off to us, and said that now I was the child's godfather.

In November of 2008 I made my first trip to Africa with Doctors Without Borders/ Medecins Sans Frontieres (MSF). Between then and February of 2012 I went on three missions with MSF, spending a total of 12 months in Africa, five months in The Sudan, three months in the Democratic Republic of Congo, and four months in Djibouti. While working in the field I sent emails home to my family and friends, generally weekly. These were meant to give an overview of my life in Africa and a description of the medical work. The experience was transformative on several levels, most importantly on a spiritual level. My stories were sent to an increasingly diverse group of people as I added "readers" after my first trip. By the third trip the emails were traveling to the United States, Switzerland, Holland, and Canada, both French and English speaking. The hardest part of being away from home for long stretches was missing the regular social gatherings that provide the fabric of life. Some of my emails include personal messages to family and friends, which I knew when sending would not be understood by all recipients. I present the emails in their original form, except for a few grammatical improvements, and have added notes as needed.

David

(Dr. David Austin)

Darfur, Sudan

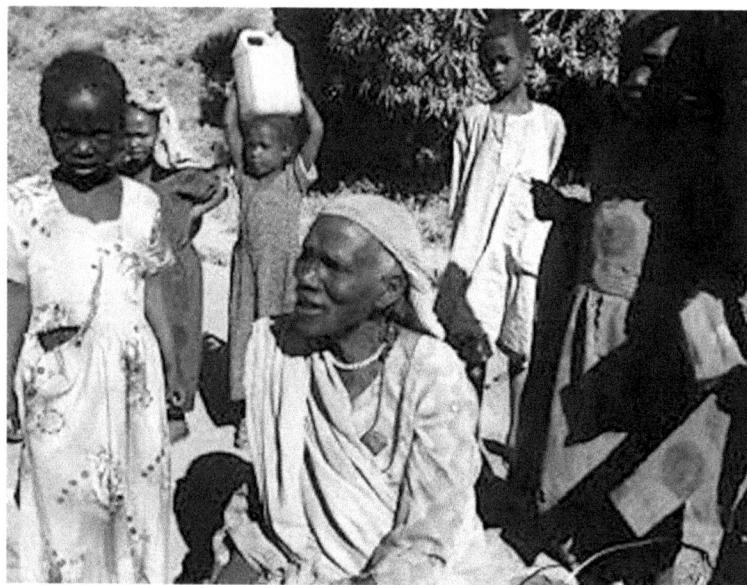

Elder and children in Darfur, met on excursion

Hello to all — as-salaam 'alaykum!!

It has been quite a remarkable trip so far, and I'll try to catch my breath for a few minutes and send off my first group message. I hope I've gotten everyone's email address in correctly. To write back to me, use the return email address and put my name in the 'subject' space.

The trip is off to a great start, with a few minor glitches. I have been in The Sudan for seven days, after two days of orientation in Geneva, Switzerland, where it was cold and rainy. I'm still a little jet lagged, but not too bad. I spent three days in Khartoum, meeting the MSF (Medecins sans Frontiers/Doctors Without Borders) staff there, and being briefed on the project here in Golo. The Khartoum staff are a most interesting international crew, several from Spain, one from Mexico, a great guy from Ethiopia, a young man with both British and US citizenship, and many nice Sudanese people. The experience for me as a visitor in the very large city (many millions) of Khartoum was most positive — many friendly people in an outdoor market, smiles and greetings galore, good food (to my exotic taste), and generally a lack of anxiety about personal safety.

Golo, however, has been surreal. The trip from Khartoum takes two days, a plane ride of about three hours to Nyala where I spent the night at the base of MSF France (I am with the Swiss branch). There I meet a 59 year old American from Chicago, a young Frenchman, and an even younger Sudanese doctor. After the night in Nyala we travelled by UN helicopter (my first helicopter ride) for about 90 minutes, making two stops on the way, arriving in Golo to be met by the MSF team plus about 25 smiling, waving, handshaking Sudanese. Quite a remarkable experience! This was yesterday. We toured the hospital and clinic here, which are very basic structures, but with enough medicines to treat the most common problems here, pneumonias, malaria, and parasites. The diagnostic tests are very basic, including a rapid test for malaria, a machine to measure hemoglobin level, and not much else. A major goal is to improve prenatal care here, mainly to get women to come in to be screened for malaria, receive prenatal vitamins, immunization against tetanus, and to be encouraged to come in to our hospital if complications occur during labor.

Today we drove the five kilometers to Killin to visit the other clinic that is part of the project here. The three mile drive took 50 minutes, roads not quite as bad as those in Haiti, only Señor Hotstream (of the people receiving this) will really know how bad that means the roads are here. Killin is a smaller medical clinic that seems to be running pretty well. I sat for some time with the Sudanese medical assistant working there, similar to a nurse practitioner or a physician's assistant in the US medical system, as he treated people with a variety of common problems (could have been at Lovejoy Health Center in Maine, except for the malaria and parasites). The most interesting part of the trip was the visit with the rebel leaders who control the area around Killin. Golo is controlled by the Sudanese government. A central goal of MSF is to be strictly impartial in providing medical care to all sides in any conflict, and that seems to be paying off here. We were greeted warmly by people, some carrying guns, who know that we are based in Golo. Though there has not been any fighting here for almost two years, both parties agree to alert MSF in advance if anything is brewing, so we can leave ahead of the trouble.

The countryside here is beautiful. We are in the mountains of Western Sudan, and it gets cool enough here at night that I have needed a blanket! During the day it is in the 80's. The mountains are quite rugged, some looking like the Dolomites. I hope to return with a lot of pictures. Unfortunately I can't send any with the emails.

I need to end soon as it is getting dark and there is no light in the room. I want to send a few personal messages.

Lois, hello to all at Lovejoy and could you forward this to Paul Forman please? No doughnuts in Sudan.

Dave Hotstream, thanks for all the trips to Haiti, I am sure they are part of the reason I am so comfortable here.

Dave Briggs, I got info on the Pats loss to Indy, but won't be able to get future news from here. Could you keep me posted on their progress and report the Celtics record and any major injuries?

If anyone is on the list by mistake let me know and I will remove.

Robert, what are you up to? Send along Cathy's email and forward this to her if you would.

Arlen, what's the latest?

Darryl, Allah must be a jazz fan (Sudan is a Muslim country) because by a series of small miracles my small keyboard made it here and I've been playing regularly so far, working on ear training also!!

Amory, I had to leave your book in Khartoum because I had too much weight for the plane, but it should be coming along in a week. I'll keep working at it. Have fun with John (but for 6 months only!). Thinking about Jen and playing 'A Child Is Born' - Send her my love and good wishes during pregnancy.

And my love and good wishes to all of you who I miss dearly. Will try to write again soon! Love, Dave Austin

Notes:

Lois is the office manager of my health center in Maine, Lovejoy. Dr. Paul Forman was my partner there. I had a habit of bringing doughnuts to work weekly.

Dave Briggs kept me posted on New England sports.

Robert and Arlen are my beloved sons, Cathy is their mother, also beloved.

Darryl was my jazz piano teacher, I played jazz weekly with Dave Briggs, Amory, and Jen, who sang with us and was pregnant at the time. John played with the group while I was gone.

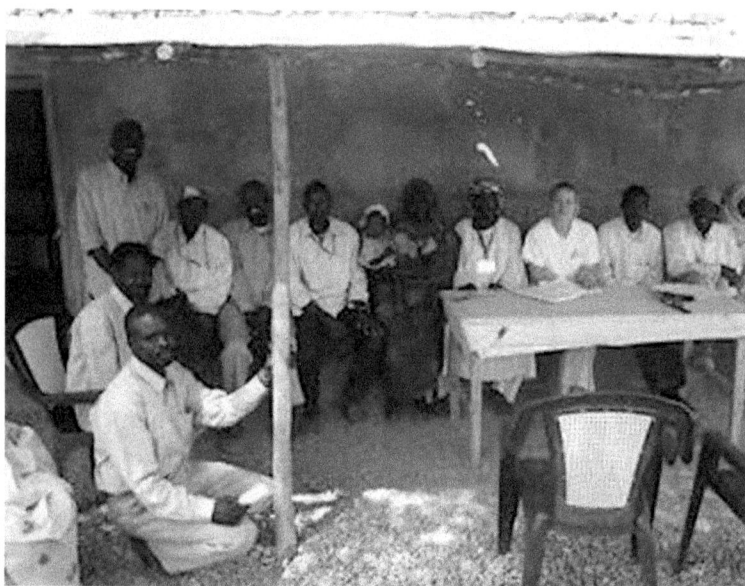

Staff in Killin

Hello!

All continues to go well here. The stars are remarkable as there is no manmade light, other than a couple of kerosene lanterns, after the generator goes off around 10:00 PM. Last night we (the MSF group) were all invited to a wedding celebration in Golo. We were welcomed as special guests, the Sudanese used their few English words to make us feel welcome, and as always the tea, in this case an especially tasty one with a smoky flavor reminiscent of Lapsang Soochong. There was music from a boom box, the loud and happy chatter that goes with such a gathering, and we were guided to use the appropriate Arabic words to congratulate the bride and groom. A most pleasant evening.

I made rounds today with the Sudanese doctor at the hospital here in Golo. He is pretty good I think. Most of the inpatient cases involve malaria and malnutrition. I also spent another chunk of time with a medical assistant seeing outpatients, many with colds and common aches and pains, much like my experience in the Dominican Republic, but the day ended with the transport of a 75 year old man via camel from a village on the other side of a mountain, probably an eight hour camel ride. He was wrapped into a chair which was bound to the camel, beside the driver. Was he suffering from an exotic tropical disease? No, he was unable to urinate, likely due to an enlarged prostate, and was on his way to receive a catheter when I left.

One of the Sudanese workers at the hospital had studied French at the university in Khartoum and was anxious to speak with me. We are on about the same level, reasonable conversational skills. He is from Golo, and his extended family lives here. After work we walked to his home, which took about 30 minutes. On the way we stopped for tea at his uncle's home. He wanted me to stay for dinner, maybe spend the night, but I made a date for dinner in the future. I had lunch today with the Sudanese medical staff who work for MSF. They are all from other parts of Sudan, most from Khartoum. They, like us westerners, are living away from their families, in a compound in Golo very similar to ours, except that judging from the meal they have a better cook! I will welcome another invitation! We ate in the traditional Sudanese fashion, communally, using pieces of bread to take food from common bowls.

I'm going to end for now and go help cook dinner.

Again, a couple of personal notes.

If anyone hears from either of my sons I would like to hear from them.

The emails intended for Beth and Ken at Shadow bounced back, so could someone send the two emails along to them, please? For anyone new to the mailing list, if you want to write me put my name in the 'subject' area. Thanks to those who have written! Poochie, could you send me the breakdown of the newly elected House and Senate—thanks!

Again, my love to you all, Dave

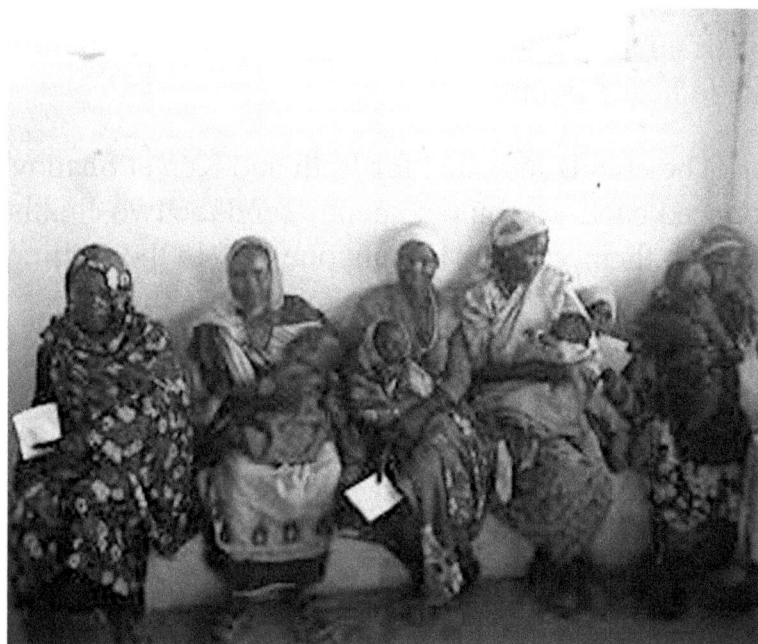

Awaiting vaccinations, Golo hospital

Sent: Friday, November 14, 2008
Subject: More news from Sudan

Hello to all!

I just spent the morning making rounds in the hospital, for the first time by myself. I had been making them with Dr. Alteib, the Sudanese doc, but today being Friday, the only day off in the Sudanese week (yes, we work full days Saturday and Sunday), and with religious significance, Alteib (his first name) asked if I was willing to make rounds alone while he went to the mosque. It was an amazing experience.

I visited the patients with a local translator, a sweet man named Mohammed Ibrahim. All of the people in the hospital speak Fur, the local language. I had Mohammed teach me greetings and such in Fur, and made quite a show (as many of you can imagine) of greeting everyone, especially the mothers with their malnourished children. They all thought it was quite hilarious, and also a good thing, to see this old white guy speaking their language, or at least trying! I may abandon my study of Arabic, or at least try to diversify.

It was most invigorating to be working independently here as a doctor for the first time. I felt right at home. The lack of technology suits me, as we do not lack good treatments for the common problems, but practically all of the diagnostic work is clinical. On my own I felt comfortable playing with the babies and engaging with their mothers. The African doctoring approach is pretty formal, though Alteib is a very friendly young man of about 30 years I would guess.

Presently there is a young man in the hospital who suffered a severe head injury after falling from a tree about a month ago. He is doing poorly and will probably die soon. During our end of week staff meeting we had an interesting discussion about his treatment. He is in a coma, developing severe bed sores, receiving intravenous fluids and tube feedings, has been treated for pneumonia, and now is receiving antibiotics for probable sepsis from the bedsores. The discussion revolved around how much further treatment he should receive. Alteib feels strongly, as do all of the Sudanese staff, that we need to continue all of the treatments we have, though all agree his condition is dire. I was not interested in trying to change his mind, in fact I felt obliged to agree with him, and given the context here I think I do agree with him. Some of the MSF staff wanted to back off on the treatment. Universal discussion.

Another universal is that all babies cry when doctors and nurses try to listen to their lungs. I asked Mohammed to point this out to one of the mothers!

Other patients in the hospital include an older woman with pneumonia, one with malaria, one I can't remember, and a couple children with both malaria and pneumonia. Most of the inpatients are malnourished children, with or without malaria, pneumonia, or dysentery, and I spent most of my morning with them. We have 10 children in the hospital, with room for maybe 16 or so. There is also one woman in labor, but I will not be involved unless it becomes complicated, as there is always a midwife available ('always' at present, that is, with our full staff here). Most women have their babies at home with traditional birth attendants. There is reportedly a very high rate of infant and maternal mortality. I am sure you can find statistics online if you are interested. The babies born at our hospital are immunized, though measles vaccine had not been available recently. Tetanus really exists here.

The man who came in by camel died overnight. He never improved though he received potentially helpful treatment with fluids and antibiotics. He possibly had prostatic or some other cancer. I gave my condolences to his large family who were present. He was 75 years which is very old for Sudan, as the life expectancy for men is my age, 54 years, and a rousing 57 years for women.

Enough medicine, this is my day off!

The shower here is great. There is warm water from a solar system and the roof is open. As the only morning person in our group I have no competition for a morning shower under the fading stars — quite fabulous! There are many trees here I do not recognize, most fairly small, about 15 feet tall, leafy, shade providers. There are six or seven of these in the courtyard of our compound. Just outside the main door lives an immense tree with a trunk four feet or more in diameter, perhaps 60 feet tall with a fully leaved top about 60 or 70 feet wide, big like the oak trees in Florida. There is lovely birdsong much of the time. Unfortunately Smoky isn't here to identify them all. I have seen several relatives of Mona (Arlen's African dove).

My travels in the Caribbean prepared me for the early morning sounds of the rooster, but not for the frequent braying of the donkeys who are commonly used for transportation here, and are tied close to my room for the night. It is quite a racket if you have yet to hear one! At first it affected my sleep, but now it is like living next to the train after the period of accommodation. There is also the call to prayer every morning and evening, a lovely singing that is quite soothing. No need for an alarm clock with the call around 5:45 am. I think I recognized the camel's voice during the night. Someone here described the sound as a cross between the voices of donkey and cow, not an unpleasant sound to my ear (unlike the donkey!).

I guess I will close for now, and thank you all for the messages! I try to send a brief individual reply when I can.

Love to you all!! Dave

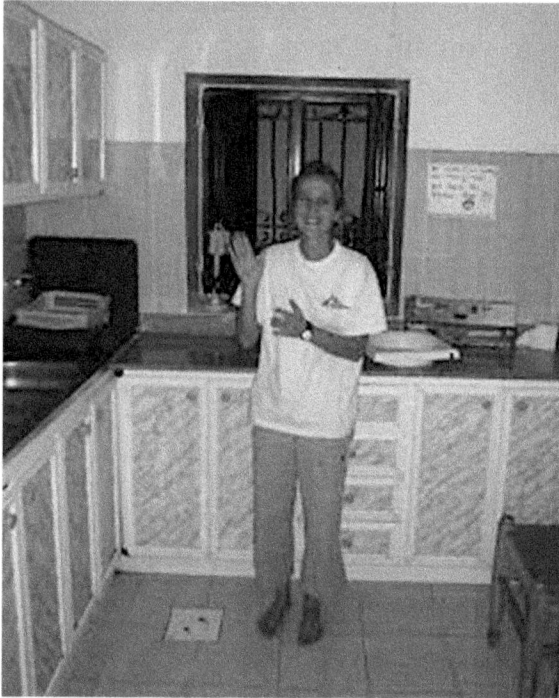

Nurse Tanya from Luxembourg

Hello to All!

Nobody said it would all be fun and exciting, and guess what, it isn't. Several hours after I wrote my last missive, on the day off, our MSF midwife asked me if I could go and investigate a reported emergency in the maternity ward, as she was in the process of having her hair braided and hoped to continue such on her only day off. On the way to the hospital I met one of the local midwives heading toward our compound, asking where our midwife was. She was clearly concerned when I said I was coming, then she was able to explain to me that there was a woman whose baby was partly out, and had been so for some time. I quickly retreated and informed our midwife that she would be accompanying me, and she agreed!

It turned out that a woman who was carrying twins had partially delivered the first baby at home, several hours earlier. The baby was breech (feet first) and had died long before she came to us. We were able to complete the delivery of the dead baby, then attended to the twin still inside. This baby was breech also. To our great relief and joy the second baby was born alive, and is doing well. It was remarkable, and seemed very appropriate, that great joy was expressed by the mother and midwives at the live birth, and little attention paid to the baby who had died. One reads and knows about infant and maternal mortality in the developing world, but it is something else to witness. Practically every mother here who has delivered several babies has lost one or two of them.

The next day (I had wisely gone to bed early, around 9:30 pm) I was soundly sleeping when, at 1:30 am, I was awoken by the sound of my name outside of the room. At first I was sure I was dreaming, but no such luck. Our midwife was calling me to join her to help with a problem, again a partially delivered breech baby who had died. The baby was premature also, and it was clear from the appearance that the baby had died some days before, while still inside the mother. I delivered the baby, tried (and I think succeeded) to express my sorrow that her baby had died, and was thanked by the mother.

So two of three babies died, but two of two mothers lived, so the present score is 3-2 in favor of the good. This is actually the thought that occurred to me at 2:30 am as I was heading back to bed. Intellectually this was a somewhat comforting thought, and I truly believed that I would be able to return to sleep with this in mind. Without consciously feeling sad or even thinking about what I had just experienced, I started sobbing in a way I have rarely experienced. Not much sleep that night.

Enough medical news! The next day while traveling to Killin a small monkey, about the size of a small cat, with a grey face, crossed in front of us on the road. Aside from this creature I have seen several squirrels. Another nighttime noise is the howling of wild dogs. As the moon wanes the stars appear brighter.

I was the only one to go to Killin yesterday (usually our nurse goes too), so at lunch time, which everyone here calls breakfast, since it is the first meal of the day (people eat 2 meals daily here), I was served food by myself. The cook actually told my translator that he should eat with me because it would not be good for me to eat alone. He was busy, so after I ate some of the meal prepared for me, I picked up my remaining food and carried it to the area where the cook, cleaner, driver, local Killin nurse, and later the translator ate. We had a good time, with a lot of laughing and joking. The people here take advantage of every opportunity to laugh and smile, quite a contrast to the picture of the part of their lives I sketched above.

Thanks again for all your messages.

Darryl, I'm starting on Anthropology in another key, listening to Clifford Brown and of course Bill Evans — helps the spirit!

Love to all, Dave

Hello!

The news about the babies here generated a lot of questions. One of Carol's co-workers, Heron, told her that the infant mortality rate overall for Africa is about 20 percent, and Carol wondered why it was so much higher here. I do not know the statistics, but it probably is not higher here, it's just that nobody calls the doctor for a normal, healthy birth. Yesterday I heard that a woman was in labor, so I hung around the maternity area and was rewarded by the sight of a beautiful newborn girl. They keep a book in the hospital where births are recorded, and I would say that the infant mortality rate for the cases that made it to the hospital was under 10 percent, maybe closer to 5 percent during this period. Still most babies born in this area are born at home, so who knows what the stats are there. Talking with people about their families, most everyone has experienced the death of two or more children for every seven or eight living, but this is not much of a scientific sample!

Thursday (yesterday) is the big market day in Golo, when people come from far and wide to sell things. My friend Nasser Aldin, who I described earlier as the only French speaking Sudanese in Golo, took me out for coffee (very good local brew with an interesting spice of some kind, maybe ginger). I met his father who runs a small shop, his mother, brother, and several aunts and uncles. We saw many of the Sudanese who work for MSF, both at the hospital and at our compound, shopping at the market, and they were pleased, and I think a little surprised, to see me there. A very fun afternoon and day in general.

Today is my day off and the Sudanese doc is rounding in the hospital. I don't have any special plans, but may go for a walk into the hills that are close by.

Yesterday being the big market day, and the day when malnourished children who are well enough to be treated outside of the hospital come in for a check-up and to receive supplemental food, we had a day of immunizations for the children. About 50 appeared with their beautiful, colorfully clad mothers, who carry their children in cloth wraps on their backs. This was truly a lovely sight, and yet another sign of the universal love and caring of parents for their children. We gave vaccinations against measles, polio, tetanus, hepatitis B, diphtheria, and pertussis (the last five combined in 1 shot!). So all in all a very good day!

Hope all is tamam (good in the Fur language) with you all

— Love, Dave

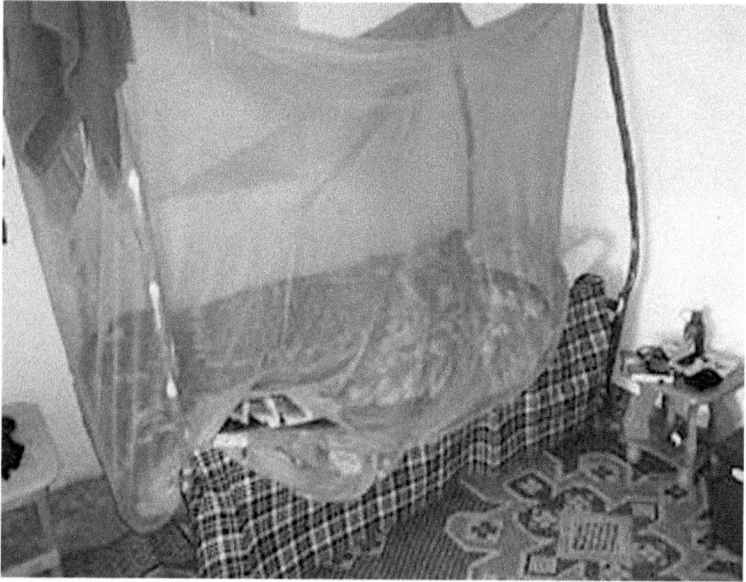

My bed in Darfur

Hello to All!

I guess I'll start with the good news. The moon is a lovely waning crescent that sits like a smile here in the early morning. With its waning the stars are the most vibrant I have ever seen, another layer behind the common constellations.

When I was in Killin yesterday, examining a small baby boy, he launched a strong stream of urine in my direction, much to the amusement of all present. I told my friend and translator Jamal that the baby was aiming at him and I blocked for him. We all had a good laugh. Of course I have experienced such humbling experiences at home, even with my own beloved children when they were of a similar age.

As I believe I wrote earlier, there is conflict

here between the government and rebel groups. When the hospital reopened last May an ambulance was provided by an international group, but was commandeered by the military, for its "protection" they said. Soldiers use it as they please, never as an ambulance. Today someone, probably the local rebel group, took possession of the ambulance. We were in our operating room, successfully (at least for the moment) saving the life of a woman whose uterus had ruptured (first I've seen in my career). While we were operating the government troops were shooting at the ambulance as it was driven into the countryside. They then came to our compound demanding to use one of our vehicles to give chase to the ambulance. Our field coordinator, Damien, refused their request, but they insisted, somewhat belligerently, and ultimately they took one of our land rovers. A short time later they returned our vehicle with a sort of apology, leading Damien to believe that things might be okay, but they soon returned, again demanding the vehicle. As a consequence we will have to leave here tomorrow, at least for awhile, much to my chagrin.

I was scheduled to return to Khartoum in six days to go through the bureaucratic hassle of getting some sort of work permit, and was expecting to be stuck there for a couple weeks, so it may work out that I will be able to do what I need to do there, then return here as planned. In any case, the hospital will not be functioning very well for the immediate future, as all of the MSF staff, including the Sudanese doctor, will be leaving.

That was the bad news. My reports will be on hold for now. I will be able to receive mails at this address I am told, and will try to keep you posted!!

Hoping for the best!

Love, Dave

Note: MSF needs to maintain neutrality wherever the organization works. The act of the Sudanese military using our vehicle for military purposes prompted our immediate departure.

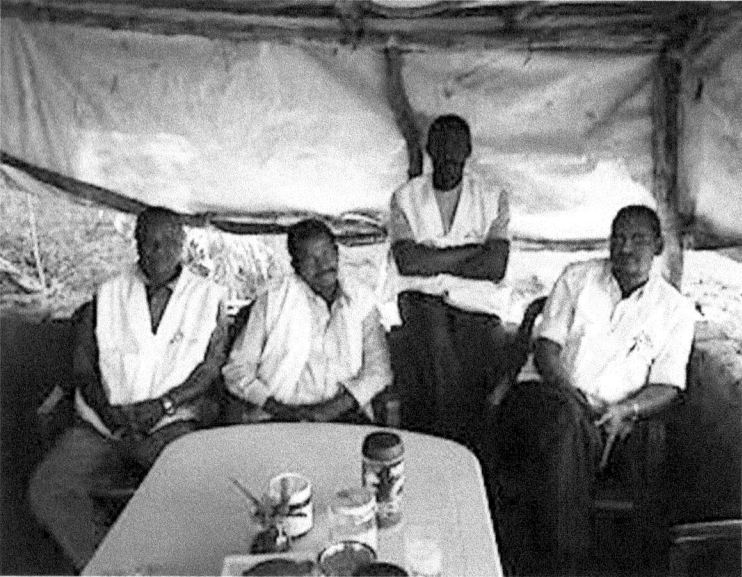

Sudanese medical staff in Golo, Dr. Altaieb on right.

Sent: Sunday, January 11, 2009
Subject: Back in Golo!

Hello!

After an interminable six weeks in Khartoum, we thankfully returned to Golo at 10:00 am today. What a warm and heartfelt greeting we received from our many friends here! The hospital has been quite busy today, and I have never felt happier to return to work.

The time in Khartoum was always interesting and often rewarding. I now have a considerable group of Sudanese friends there, and a number of international friends. I spent a lot of time with a Chinese woman, Wang Ya, who is the only Chinese national I have ever met. She is quite proud of her country, and after many fascinating discussions with her I understand why. She describes a culture rich with communal caring, proud of many thousands of years of accomplishments, and understanding of some of its faults.

I met two great characters from Austria, one a young doctor and the other a committed nihilist, both lovely people.

I spent a good deal of time with Isaac Juma, a man from South Sudan who I met during our exit from here back in November. He is a medical assistant for MSF France, having worked with them for almost 10 years. He suffered a mild heart attack in the field, and was evacuated to Khartoum for medical care, and I was asked to accompany him and tend to him medically for the day we were together in Nyala. I visited him daily while he was in the hospital in Khartoum. There I met his wife and youngest child. Later in my stay they invited me to their home on the outskirts of Khartoum where I met his 3 older children and his friend Dixon Sadikimbegha, a real character from Tanzania. Reida Kolo, Isaac's wife, cooked a fabulous seven-course traditional African meal for us, enough for at least ten people, and they tried to get me to finish it all. I did my best, which as some of you know is pretty good, but there was still a bit left at the end!

I had malaria while in Khartoum, not an especially bad case. I had been taking the preventive medicine Larium, which needless to say is not 100%

effective. I made the diagnosis quite quickly, started treatment, and felt pretty good after about 10 days.

It really feels like home here in Golo. We had been here long enough to know our way around, be comfortable with the local staff, and generally feel useful. A pigeon has moved into the eave of the porch in front of my room, and it looks like a smaller bird is nesting somewhere on the porch also, two good omens.

For those of you receiving your first email from me, to respond use the email address and put my name in the 'subject' space.

I am writing now on the evening of the 10th of January. I plan to add a bit in the morning, then hit 'send'. First a bit of housekeeping.

Dave Briggs, I know all too well about the shaft that the Patriots got, the Celtics mini-slump (but how did they do against Cleveland?), the Sox signing Rocco (good move I think) and Smoltz, but from this day forward, till further notice, please resume sending the sports updates which have been much appreciated.

I am expecting a birth announcement sometime next month.

Happy birthday to Zoro on the 17th (in case I forget).

More to come in the morning...

Now it is 7:00 am here. I got up at 5:00 am, my old routine, studied the beautiful sky with practically full moon hence somewhat diminished stars, still far superior to Khartoum's constant haze and ambient light. Tried to listen to the BBC to hear about the International Criminal Court's (ICC) expected indictment of Sudan's President Bashir, something that has been expected for the past several months, but which may finally happen soon, and may make things again more difficult for western organizations trying to work in Sudan.

I was called back to the hospital in the evening to see a one year old who did not seem especially ill, and a young man with cerebral malaria who was plenty sick. I will learn in an hour or so whether I was correct about the former and able to help the latter.

It was good to hear the donkeys again during the night. There was a strong wind from time to time, and the temperature is about 50 degrees Farenheit at present. If yesterday is typical it will be about 80 degrees by midday.

Well, it is good to be back at the computer in Golo.

I hope you are all well.

Siempre, Dave

Hello to all!

There is much good news to report, which is always nice! The young man with malaria is doing well. I took his picture yesterday sitting with his father, smiling. He is still a little jaundiced and tired, but appears to be on the way to full recovery, and will probably go home today. While he was very sick he appeared much older than he does now. I had guessed he was in his early twenties, but now I would say 15 years or so.

About 36 hours ago, around 9:00 pm, I was called to the hospital to see a child in the malnutrition unit. A thirteen month old girl, now weighing 13 pounds, she had been in the hospital for 10 days under treatment for pneumonia. During the day she had appeared well, gaining a little weight, with no obvious problems. Earlier in the week, the same night that the youngster with malaria was so ill, I was asked to see another child also, and now I think it was this same little girl, who at that time was receiving antibiotics (ceftriaxone for the medically inclined) and was doing quite well. I could not figure out why the nurses had called me then, as she seemed vigorous, and like all tykes her age wanted little to do with me as she was trying to sleep. The recent return visit was a far different story. The child appeared very close to death—lethargic, eyes half opened, fever, very rapid heartbeat, shallow breathing—she did not respond in the slightest to the two injections she received in her muscles.

Needless to say I was shocked by her appearance, but add to this the reality that no one there could speak any meaningful English (it was the night crew, during the day there would have been a translator and many of the day staff speak English reasonably well). My few words of Arabic and Fur were not impressing anyone, and everyone was appropriately concerned about the baby. After a few moments of trying to take some sort of 'history' (like when did the child become ill) I woke up and went off with one of the nutritional assistants to get antibiotics stored in another part of the hospital. The child received doses of ceftriaxone and gentamycin 15 minutes after my arrival, pretty good by US standards! I stayed there with the child, family, and staff for about an hour, not that I had anything else 'medical' to offer, and as the child did not seem to be getting any worse, I left.

I hoped it was a good sign that I wasn't called again during the rest of the night, though I also considered that they might not have wanted to awaken me with news of the child's death, and when I spoke with the guards at our compound in the morning (they would have been called by walkie talkie to fetch me if needed during the night), 'spoke' using sign language and my few words, they assured me that the child was tamam (very good). She was being fed by her mother when I saw her during morning rounds, and drinking from a cup by herself later in the day. I also took a nice picture of her with her mother (in her recovered state only).

The rapid recovery of very ill children, when illness is due to bacterial infection (and is treated), is something everyone who cares for children quickly learns about, but this case impressed me as much as any I have ever seen, from a purely medical point of view, as I have never seen a sicker appearing child. This includes a two-year old who I cared for in the emergency room during my residency, septic with meningococcus (a very lethal bug), who also received antibiotics within about 15 minutes, but who died several days later.

More good news. The pigeon who has been sitting under the roof of my porch is sitting on a couple eggs. I hope that my presence does not interfere with her reproduction. I have named her

"Pidgy" in memory of an old bird friend of mine, Gully, who you see from the name was a bird of a different feather.

Some mixed news. My toy piano is on the fritz. Yesterday it stopped working entirely. It had shown some signs of impending failure, as the volume control had occasionally failed to work, but previously had recovered with some jiggling. I should note that this instrument, a Roland made in Japan (much to the pleasure of my friend and co-worker Toshihero), has been a great investment, costing about $90 ten years ago. It helped me learn jazz piano during breaks at my job at Lovejoy, spent some time on loan in Sudbury, and otherwise provided excellent service. When it quit this time I removed the bottom of the case, revealing all the inscrutable microchip technology, and also revealing that the mechanism related to the volume control was not reachable without removing everything, which I was sure would be lethal for the machine. I closed it up, then hacked out a small opening around the volume control. Now, if I blow air into the area where the control is (like artificial respiration) the crazy machine works for a few minutes, then fades away, until given a few more breaths. If I can nurse it along like this for the next three months I will be happy, and even if I can't I won't complain.

Love to all, David

Sent: Monday, January 19, 2009
Subject: Another day (or two)

Hello!

All is quite well here, and a few interesting things to report.

Carol told me there was supposed to be a meteor shower this past weekend, so I was quite excited, with the clarity of the night sky here, hoping for a great show. Perhaps (I know so little about astronomy) one had to be in the northern hemisphere to see a lot, but I spent a great couple of hours lying on my back on the warm earth watching the stars. I thing I saw a couple shooting stars. This morning, in my warm, open-roofed shower, I was making a mental note on how to describe the appearance of the Big Dipper as viewed from the shower. I swear I am not making this up, at the time of my shower the dipper is oriented precisely in a fashion to be pouring water on me! As I was admiring the stars this morning a brilliant shooting star travelled across the dipper's handle.

For the past two days I have been the only medical person at our 'satellite' clinic in Killin. The regular medical assistant there, Zachariah, developed malaria and had to miss a day, and reportedly his father is very ill, so Zachariah has gone to be with him in a nearby village. A subplot is that he may have not had any sort of vacation for years, and may be taking advantage of this opportunity to take a break. I certainly wouldn't blame him! So for the past two days I have cared for the 70 or so patients he sees each day. This has been mainly great fun for me, seeing many women with babies and young children, most not too sick (just like at home), all mothers worried about their children (just like at home), great senses of humor, smiles all around. So Lois, before you start thinking about future increased productivity at Lovejoy, a few words about the nature of medical care here.

At Killin we have only three tests available, and the rapid test for malaria is the only one we use regularly. My medical record documentation involves scribbling a few words (I love it!!). Though we have a good number of quality medicines, the options available to treat the diseases we commonly see (malaria, skin infections, pneumonia) are few, so there is no need to spend a lot of time pondering what tests to order, whether a referral is needed, etc. So to see a patient every five minutes of so is relatively easy.

Midway through my afternoon of work yesterday,

shortly after speaking with Carol on the satellite phone while all the people, or I should say all the men, working with me were praying, a woman of about 60 years was brought in by her family. She needed help to walk and appeared very ill. The history was that she had been well until four days ago when she developed fever and sweats at night, and had gotten progressively weaker. She also had headache and body pains but was thinking clearly according to her family, and was still able to eat and drink. She did not have a fever when I saw her, but her pulse was 120 and respiratory rate 56. As we doctors are taught in medical school, the history leads to the diagnosis 90% of the time, and I have been here long enough to have malaria on the top of the diagnosis list much of the time, even without fever. I was a bit surprised that the family did not tell me that she had malaria, because until yesterday every patient who came in saying they had malaria were proved correct by our test, whether or not they appeared ill or had fever. The first exception was a younger man with no symptoms, whose self-diagnosis was contradicted by our test. The woman's test was positive, we started treating her at Killin, then brought her back to the hospital in Golo at the end of the day (after a house call on the way back to see a younger handicapped man who probably has pneumonia) to spend a couple days in the hospital, assuming all goes well.

Needless to say it was a busy day, and that got me into a bit of trouble. I was the only one at Killin from our group, which is unusual. We carry a satellite phone to communicate with the team at Golo, and I generally let whoever else is there perform this duty. I called Damien, our good field coordinator, when we arrived, which is the security rule, and when I called him again around 5:30 pm to say we were ready to come back I was unpleasantly surprised to find him very upset with me. I had completely forgotten that I was supposed to call at 3:30 pm if I was going to be there later than that, and as I was carrying the phone in my pocket (the phone needs to be outside to reach the satellites) he had been unable to reach me for two hours.

This lack of contact activated security rules requiring him to call our big boss in Khartoum, and he was on the verge of starting out to look for me, so no surprise he was upset. I misunderstood what he was saying to me on the phone to mean he had called the big boss to discuss my imminent firing for the breach of protocol, so I was much relieved to find him in good spirits and accepting of my apologies on my return. Knowing how hard it can be to avoid misunderstandings among people who share the same language, culture, etc., you can imagine the potential for miscommunication and misunderstanding when dealing with people from different cultures, none of whom share a native tongue.

Well, that is plenty for now. Enjoy the Maine winter, unless you are lucky enough to be on Sanibel Island at the moment!

Siempre, Dave

Sent: Saturday, January 24, 2009

Subject: Starting a new week in Golo

Hello,

It is just after 6:30 am on Saturday morning, and with the call to prayer in the background, I am thinking about the start of the workweek, which is NOW. I have been in Sudan for about three months, but after a lifetime of loving Saturday and Sunday mornings it is still a bit of a shock when my watch tells me it is Saturday and I am off for a full day of work. Friday is the one day off in the week here in Golo, and since I share the hospital work and coverage for emergencies with only one other doctor, yesterday was the first day off I have had during the 2 weeks of our return. Many of the working days are not especially busy, but the modern western mind likes to have a couple days off at the end of the week. In the big city of Khartoum things are a bit more western, with many people having both Friday and Saturday off, but not so here in the countryside!

Yesterday three of us took a fabulous hike in the morning, starting off when the air was still cool, maybe 65 degrees, and returning after four hours, around 1:00 pm, in dry 90 degree heat. Our guide was my friend and translator Mohammed Ibrahim, who wanted to show us a waterfall. This might seem relatively commonplace in many places, but here in Golo, as in Khartoum, everything in parched, dusty, hot—one always feels fine dust in the mouth (which may help dental care by acting like pumice when brushing). So talk of waterfalls seemed very fanciful, and Mohammed had also told us that some of the larger waterfalls were 'turned off' at present, as they only exist during the rainy season.

After walking for an hour in the usual dry, dusty environment, we suddenly came upon a small stream where many people were fetching water. Now I know what an oasis looks like. We followed the stream to its source, a walk of about half an hour. The stream banks were surrounded by lush, green gardens, mainly growing scallions and garlic at present. We saw tomatoes from an earlier harvest drying in the ever present sun. I was given a scallion to eat, and it was truly the sweetest and juiciest I have ever tasted. There were mango and orange trees galore growing along the stream, trees filled with birds, and we saw many beautiful dragonflies, red and blue ones, more vividly colored than the lovely ones which inhabit Maine. We met several people who work in the hospital in Golo, who were pleased that we were visiting their village, Sari Sam it is called. Quite the refreshing change from the Golo scene!

Now I look forward to 13 days of work, the first seven on call, before my next 'weekend'!

Two days ago I suffered a period of depression when my piano stopped working entirely for 24 hours, but with the rest and renewed resuscitation efforts it revived. Daryl, my piano teacher, will be the ultimate judge of this, but I felt I was playing with a special intensity and improved quality when I received my reprieve from what I feared would be a three month sentence without my precious toy piano.

A truck arrived a couple days ago with supplies for the hospital and some food for us. We were (some of us in any case) excited by certain foods not obtainable here: canned tuna, mayonnaise, jam, cereal in a box, Pringles potato chips (two small cans), Nutella (yuk), some good coffee (hurray), olive oil, and a few other items that clearly did not make a big impression on me. I was more concerned, regarding food, when we had some oranges last week that were not so good, quite tasteless. Happily the last batch is great. My ritual is to eat one each morning, a hangover perhaps from the days when my mother insisted I drink orange juice every morning.

So there you have it, life goes on here.

Still expecting a birth announcement in the next

month. Wondering about the latest sports news.

On that note, I listened to Obama take the oath, deliver his speech, then heard interviews from Kogelo, Kenya, the village his father came from. There was a big party there, and some enterprising soul had been marketing Senator Obama Beer, which needless to say was most popular on the occasion (per BBC report), and had almost run out, but they were sending out for more!

Hope all is well where you are!

Love from Golo, Dave

Sent: Friday, January 30, 2009
Subject: Short Weekend

Hello!

Well, it is Friday morning here, the 'weekend', and the last day of my week on call. What a relief. The week has been busy with too much excitement at night, translate as not enough sleep for me, and I have had a cold, adding a bit of insult to injury, as my mother would have said.

It has gotten a bit warmer here, or to be more precise, it does not cool down as much during the night, while the daytime temperature stays around 90. Still it is cool enough to sleep comfortably at night. The moon is a crescent and the stars continue to shine brightly, though occasionally there are clouds in the morning, a sign of the slow transition to the season of rain, which generally does not arrive in full till the end of March.

Medically the week on call began with an evening arrival, Saturday, of a pregnant woman with a prolapsed umbilical cord, and consequently a baby who had already died. The remaining problem was that this was her first pregnancy, her cervix was three centimeters dilated and she was not in labor, and she is a tiny woman. I hoped for her sake to be able to deliver the baby vaginally, but after an optimistic beginning where, with Pitocin, she progressed to full dilatation, a couple hours of pushing without progress, and several attempts to help with our vacuum forceps, we concluded that she would not deliver vaginally, and proceeded to perform a C- section, which went very smoothly. My legs were aching at the end of all this!

Early Monday morning, 2:00 am, I was roused to see a young pregnant woman who had been in the hospital a couple days with a urinary tract infection. I had not seen her before, as my colleague had admitted her and reportedly she was doing well. They called me because she had developed severe abdominal pain, and she looked quite ill when I arrived. Her belly was mildly distended and she appeared very pale. The Sudanese doc has a bad habit of treating many people with antispasmodics, medicines intended to help with cramping, but which also inhibit the normal action of the bowel, and he continues these medicines for a long time at high doses. I thought this might be the source of her pain, so I stopped the medicine and gave her pain medicine and i.v. fluids. In the morning (the soonest the test could be done) we learned that her hemoglobin was three (normal being around 12), so she has been severely anemic for some time, but not symptomatic from this. There probably are many reasons for her anemia, but our extensive testing revealed that she did not have malaria (at present). We gave her blood transfusions from her relatives, as we are able to do blood typing. This did not explain her abdominal pain, which unfortunately continued. I hypothesized that slowing her bowel with the medication allowed undesirable bugs to proliferate, bugs that did not mind the antibiotic she was receiving (Giardia for example, which everyone has here), so I tried giving her treatment for this possibility, and as of this afternoon she is much improved. Hoping for one happy ending for now.

Later that day there was some comic relief, for me at least, when I was faced that the problem of a young boy who had stuck a large seed deep into his ear. With the help of several strong men holding the child, I was able to remove the seed, using a small forceps and a cheap otoscope. As some of you know, in my previous practices I rather pride myself on being able to remove unwanted objects from children's noses and ears. It did not take long for my reputation to spread here, for two days later, with similar tools, I removed a larger seed from the nose of a smaller girl. I am saving these seeds as evidence.

In between these happier moments there was another obstetrical disaster. A 30 year old woman showed up after laboring for the day in a distant village with her seventh child. She has three living children from these seven pregnancies, and the seventh was not lucky. She had reached full dilatation several hours earlier, pushed for awhile, then contractions stopped. The baby had died by her arrival here. With some difficulty I was able to deliver the baby, using the vacuum forceps. We also had a very malnourished baby die in the hospital, so all in all not a very happy week.

The combination of lack of sleep and a truly mild cold has me missing the comforts of home more that I had been. The instant coffee with powdered milk suddenly does not taste as good, not to mention missing a cold Shipyard, or a Guinness for that matter (by the way, Dave, are the Celtics still playing and have the Sox signed Barry Bonds?).

Well, it is off to the hospital, then one more day and night, then back to work tomorrow and for six more days (but peaceful nights!), then the beloved 'weekend' to look forward to.

Enjoy your weekend! Love, Dave

Sent: Friday, February 6, 2009
Subject: Another week

Hello to All!!

It has been a very busy week here work wise, many people, mostly children, sick enough to be in the hospital, some appearing near death on arrival, and all living at this moment to the best of my knowledge, not having been to the hospital yet this morning, after sleeping peacefully through the night as my Sudanese colleague covered things. Most of those hospitalized have malaria, often complicated by pneumonia, but we have had a couple meningitis cases. We cannot identify the type of meningitis, but the youngster I admitted was very ill, likely from the bacterial meningitis that is so potentially lethal. There is an epidemic of meningococcal meningitis in Southern Sudan (far from here geographically and politically) which MSF is trying to respond to, and we are hoping that we are not seeing the first signs of an epidemic here, as we have heard of several other suspected cases and relatively sudden deaths of young people from the village that the child I saw comes from.

Today the plan is for Tanya (our nurse from Luxemborg) and I to travel to this village and investigate. Headquarters in Khartoum is sending us some kits to rapidly identify the specific bacterial cause of meningitis if we find other cases. If it appears that an epidemic is starting in our area, we will try to diminish its impact with a vaccination campaign. I look forward to the 'field trip'.

On the social front, three of my friends took me out to the local market several days ago, after work. I had thought we were going for coffee or tea, which they always insist on buying for me. Mohammed Ibrahim the translator, Nasser Aldeen the French speaker, and Osman the dressing nurse were my hosts. Osman is about my age I believe, but the precise age of people here is often a mystery. Osman once told me he was 56 years old, but later chose a lower number, I think after I was joking with him about his advanced age. As we were walking to the market, there was talk about eating some meat. This was a bit distressing to me, as the meat that has been part of my meals here has been uniformly bad, except for the liver (no further comment needed), tough, grisly, cooked to death, I generally pass on it. So with some trepidation I agreed to the meat plan. Another great surprise was in store for me. We were having coffee in a restaurant run by Mohammed's wife, a lovely woman in her mid-thirties, mother of seven children, who spoke some English. Nasser excused himself, and soon returned with a bag of raw meat.

Next we moved on to another tea drinking establishment. The whole market would look like a war zone to someone not used to the buildings here, dilapidated structures of crumbling brick and rocks, with awnings made of old packaging materials, burlap or some more modern equivalent, frayed and dusty. Nasser delivered the meat to one of these businesses, and I could see men there cutting meat. Later, when we walked over to the place, we found our meat grilling on skewers over charcoal. We went into an inner room where people were seated on mats, eating. We sat down and were served our grilled meat, accompanied by a savory dipping sauce and a mixture of salt and cayenne pepper. It was delicious! I learned that the meat cost eight Sudanese pounds per kilo, about $1.50 per pound, and the cost of the preparation and condiments added another 20 cents. Not a bad deal!

The moon sets early now, and the stars are as vibrant as ever. I certainly did not know the constellations any better than the average American before coming here, and after studying them nightly, I wonder if I will be able to find them in Maine. The scorpion's curling tail is so brilliant now I am sure I wouldn't have missed it if it were nearly this visible back home, and the Gemini twins appear to be dancing across the sky here, low to the horizon. Remarkable.

Therese's Dream

Yesterday I was called on to see an eight year old girl who had been raped in a village five hours walk from here. The alleged rapist was in jail, and the child and her mother had walked here to obtain a medical statement for the court. If I had not known the story of the rape, which reportedly had occurred five days earlier, I would have thought only of meeting a most pleasant, friendly, and engaging child. This is only to describe how normal the child seemed. I do believe she was raped, a sadly familiar story of rape by someone the family knew, a relative perhaps. The child's mother was visibly upset, and it was worth it to her to walk five hours to try to do something about it.

Other than this sad story the medical news is generally good, as alluded to above, no obstetrical disasters, they are probably being saved up for my week on call, which begins tomorrow.

I hope you are all well. I am feeling well and rested. Still, I could use some sports news, David! And there should be a birth announcement any time now.

Love, Dave

Sent: Friday, February 13, 2009
Subject: Friday the 13th in Golo

Hello All!

Well, the week has been quite eventful, and I will try to pass on all the news. It is the 13th here, and I have always liked the number, a nice prime one, and have never noted any especially bad luck associated with the day. Luck is often bad here in Darfur, but as often as not some sort of 'silver lining' phenomenon seems to prevail, as perhaps you will see.

The week started with a remarkable event, a mentally ill woman in her 40's was shot by soldiers who were guarding the local market. My initial reaction was predictable outrage, how could this happen? The woman nearly died from blood loss, was cared for initially by Dr. Altaieb who was on call, kept alive by intravenous fluids, and when I met her in the morning she had a pulse of 140, blood pressure 70/50 (dangerously low), and a hemoglobin of 3.8 (severe anemia). Her temperature was low, and most thought she was dying. We found relatives of hers to donate blood, and she received two transfusions later in the day. The next day she was eating, awake, hemoglobin 8, and vital signs okay.

I learned from my friend Mohammed Ibrahim the details of the shooting. The woman is well known to be crazy. The shooting took place at 10:00 pm. No one other than the guards was in the market. This part of the world is in a low-grade civil war, and just before we had to leave a soldier was killed. The woman was walking close to the market, it was dark, a soldier told her to stop and she immediately started running away. The soldier, who could not see who she was, shot.

Two days later I helped the dressing nurse change her dressings. The silver lining is that she was not killed. First, I had never seen a gunshot wound, so had little idea what to expect. She has two 'entry wounds' in her right leg, one in the upper front of her thigh, and one higher, close to the pelvic bone. These wounds are tiny, looking like little more than small scratches that need only a bandaid and a mother's kiss. The 'exit wounds' are another story, ragged rips in the flesh, several inches in width. The one in the upper thigh looked okay, but the higher wound is close to the rectum (an inch closer and she surely would have died), larger than the first, but for now not life threatening. A bullet had also entered her right forearm, apparently after passing through her leg. The arm appears to be broken and there is no exit wound, so the bullet presumably sits inside her arm, where it will remain. My apologies to any NRA members in the audience, but my initial response was that guns are a creation of the devil. The woman is doing quite well a week later.

Two days after this we had a difficult delivery. I knew that someone was in labor and things were not going well, so around noon I checked in at maternity. Altaieb had been there trying to deliver the baby with the vacuum forceps, without success, and everyone was disappointed. When I examined the woman, who was pushing vigorously when I arrived, we were encouraged to find that the baby had descended some, though there was a lot of moulding of the baby's head (shaping of the baby's head during descent through the birth canal, suggesting a relatively difficult passage). With renewed enthusiasm the midwives encouraged the mother's efforts, and slow progress seemed to ensue. I now feel very comfortable with the midwives, and enjoy being with them at deliveries, even with the high likelihood of disaster. The laboring women are unbelievable. Of course they know nothing of pain injections or epidurals, and take the birthing process wholly in stride, often smiling and interactive between contractions and pushes. I have taken to wearing a taiga, a traditional muslim head cover, a gift from Mohammed Ibrahim. During the labor above, after checking with the midwives to be sure I was not being culturally inappropriate, I placed my taiga on the laboring woman's head, hoping to bring her good luck. Everyone had a good laugh. When I left to do some other work she seemed to

be making slow progress. Returning to check in a
bit later I met Altaieb walking away from maternity,
having just delivered a dead baby with the vacuum
forceps. I went to give my condolences.

I have been on call for the past six nights but have
only been called once, though this was a memorable
call. The night before last maternity called. The local
midwife had noted that the woman she was attending,
who was having her first baby, and had reached the
point of vigorous pushing, was showing what the
midwife thought was the baby's hand. It turned out to
be the baby's foot, resting next to its bottom. Breech
deliveries are almost always done by C-section in
the 'modern world', generally for good reason, but
this was not going to happen here. It is such a long
and complicated process to orchestrate a C-section
here that they are reserved for situations where the
mother's life is threatened. So I was on my own.

First I attempted to push the foot back inside the
mother's uterus, a recommended approach in this
situation, but was unable. The delivery proceeded
well to a point, the foot not appearing to interfere
much with progress of labor. Unfortunately, after
the baby's legs and buttocks delivered, one of the
arms was extended above the baby's head, a further
complication which added a couple extra minutes
to the delivery, extra minutes the baby did not have
to spare. I tried to resuscitate the baby, first using a
mask that was too large, then with the old mouth-
to-mouth method, but with no heartbeat I did not
continue for long. As I was repairing the episiotomy

another laboring mother came into the room (we
have two delivery tables in a relatively small room)
attended by the midwife. The woman was having her
third baby, and all was going well. I wrapped up the
dead baby, who looked very beautiful, and presented
her to her mother, initially not being sure that my
western approach was correct here, but judging by
her response as she held the baby close it was a good
thing. She was not crying as she held her baby, but she
appeared sad, accepting of her fate. Where the death
of a baby is so common—most every woman I have
asked has lost two or more babies—the loss is not the
unique tragedy it appears in the west, to be suffered
alone or in a support group, but instead appears to be
an initiation into a sisterhood of shared loss.

Later that morning when I told Mohammed about
the death of the baby he immediately asked me if
the mother was okay. When I told him she was, he
basically responded that this is good, don't worry. I
am sure I will not 'get used' to babies dying in a the
few months I will spend here. It seems to me that
while misery is doled out in small ladles in 'our'
world, and this in no way minimizes the magnitude of
our true misery, here it is distributed by the bucketful.

There was a bit of comic relief after the delivery.
While I was helping the midwife with the normal
delivery, the woman who had just undergone a
difficult delivery and lost her baby sat up at the side
of her delivery table unassisted and practically leapt
off, tripping on a trash bucket. She caught herself and
landed like a ballerina, then walked out of the room.

The meningitis scare seems to be a viral outbreak, severe enough disease to kill two children, though they died in the village without benefit of our hospital. I am two for four in lumbar puncture success, not bad considering that I cannot remember the last time I did one, but can recall vividly being taught how to do them by Dr. John Salvato, now famous pediatrician in Waterville, Maine, formerly pediatric resident in Rochester, New York where I first met him. He must have done a pretty good job, and the two failed attempts were due to extreme vigor on the part of the children, the old saying being that if the child is strong enough to prevent the spinal tap it is not needed.

My piano is hanging in there, with regular resuscitation required.

Enough for now. I am anxiously awaiting a birth announcement, having been informed by sources that Jen has had quite enough of this pregnancy, though she is still singing.

In one week I have a break, a week off, and inshallah I will be heading to Egypt to meet up with my son Robert. Needless to say I greatly look forward to this time off. Should be one more 'report' before then.

Be well! Love, Dave

Hello My Friends,

A different week for me. I spent four consecutive days at the clinic in Killin substituting for the medical assistant there who was on vacation, reportedly his first in several years. It was quite busy. The first day I saw 85 people in about six hours of work, 'slower' days brought 60 or 70. Cases ranged from the common cold to that of an older woman with such a severe oral infection (Ludwig's angina for the medical in the crowd) that she could hardly swallow or breathe. We were able to start treatment with intravenous antibiotics in Killin, then we sent her to the Golo hospital. She looked much improved when I saw her the following morning. A young man of about 14 years showed me an unusual complication of malaria, obvious blood in the urine. He was quite sick, but still able to be treated out of the hospital.

The travel back and forth on the 'road' from Golo to Killin is more like a 45 minute carnival ride than a car trip, and the adventure effects some people more than others. To my good fortune, I have no trouble with motion sickness. On an earlier trip, when our midwife Nadifa was on board, she had vomited several times in transit, including vomiting on me (only on my foot, so not too bad). I had forgotten this episode until history repeated itself as we were transporting a sick child and his mother back to Golo. The child was quite ill, but slept most of the way. The mother was fine for about half of the ride then, guess what. I was sitting next to her, trying to be of some comfort and holding closed a hole in the plastic bag she was barfing into, when it became apparent that there were other holes in the bag. Curiously, and again fortunately for me, I have never been especially offended by vomit.

My vacation plans are now on hold. The helicopter flights to this part of Darfur have been cancelled for the past week, not due to any trouble in Golo, but in other areas where the UN flies. My trip has been delayed until Wednesday, inshallah. I certainly am not counting on the vacation at this point, but it will be a big problem for us if the helicopter flights are not resumed. Even though all is peaceful here in Golo, the canceling of flights is a sign of general instability in the wider area, and we may have to leave again, of so I am told. So, for several reasons, I am hoping for a vacation next week.

The stars have been especially brilliant with the

waning moon, and my reward for studying them at some length this early morning included two shooting stars. From vomit to stars life goes on here. Sorry I lack the energy for more stories today. If you hear from me next Friday it will probably be a bad sign!

Hope all is well where you are!

Love, Dave

First Intermission

I did make it to Cairo and had several adventures there, a great visit with my son Robert, then some time scuba diving in the Red Sea, staying in a nice room on the water in Dahab for $11 per night! MSF contacted me there, letting me know that our team had been evacuated again and advising me to extend my stay in Egypt (no problem) till further notice.

I did return to Khartoum several days later, where we sequestered for another several weeks before Bashir finally threw us all out of his country. At one point a Peruvian nurse and I had tickets to fly to another part of Darfur to work in a different project. I was all packed and making my morning coffee, ready to get back to work. The knock at my door, which I expected to be my driver ready to deliver me to the airport, turned out to be my friend Sylvia from administration, telling me that 2 MSF workers at the project I was to join had been kidnapped, and our trip was off.

I returned to my old job in Maine, certain that this was not to be my only journey to Africa. My assignment to the Democratic Republic of Congo was to be my first French speaking job. In preparation I spent a week of immersion in French speaking Trois Pistoles, a small city in eastern Quebec Province, Canada.

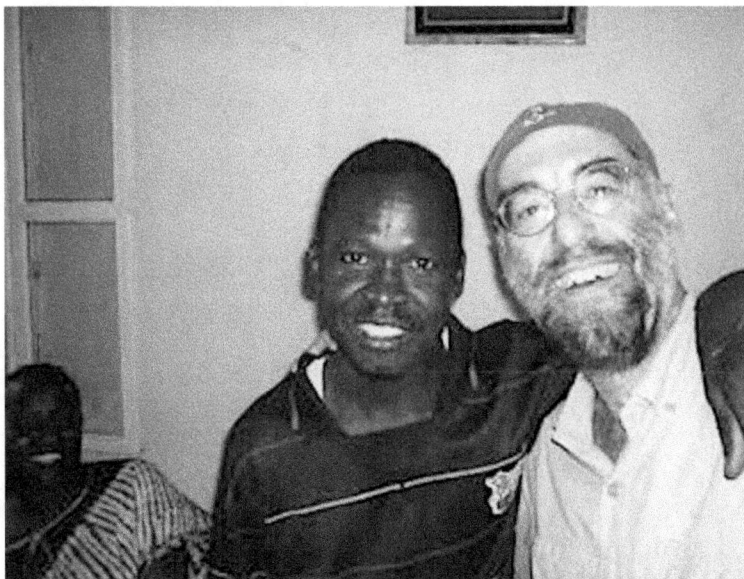

Dr. Austin with his friend Isaac from South Sudan

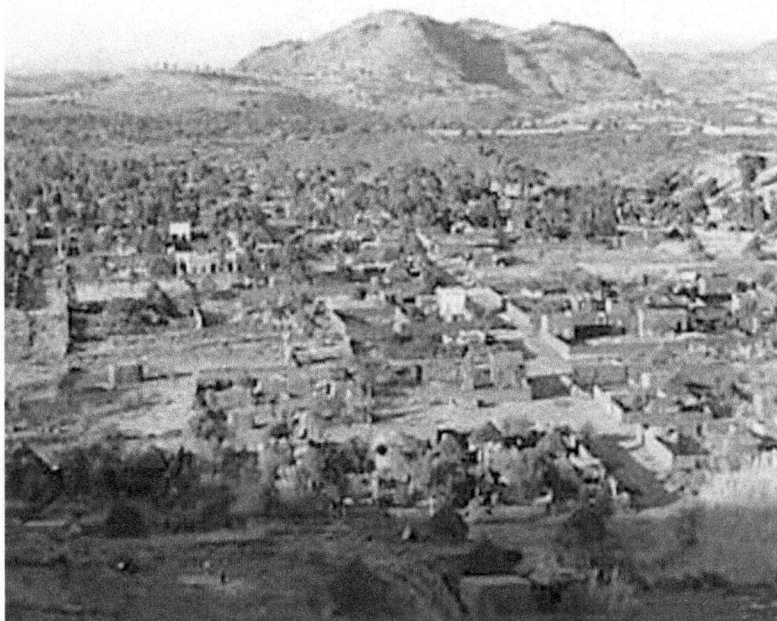

Village of Golo

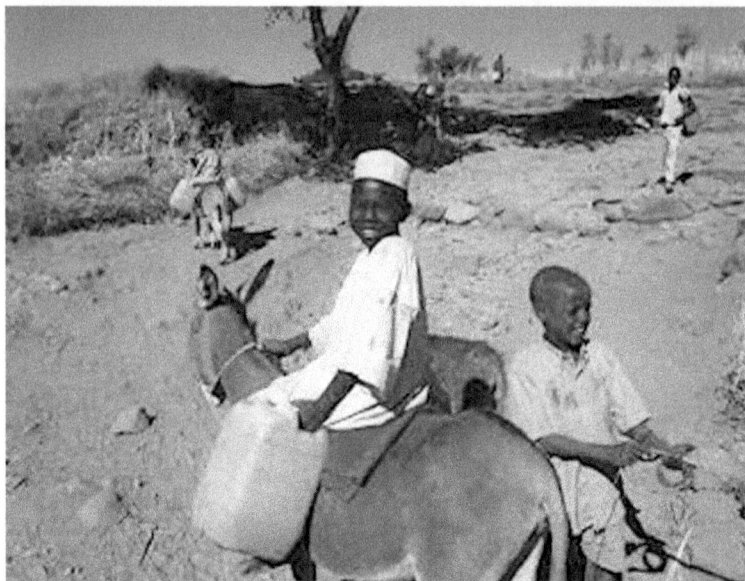

Excursion

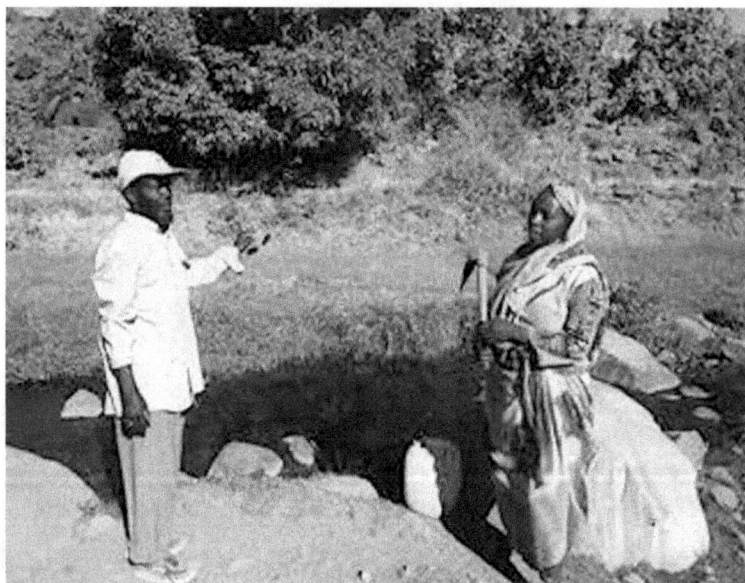

Excursion, met woman who also worked at hospital

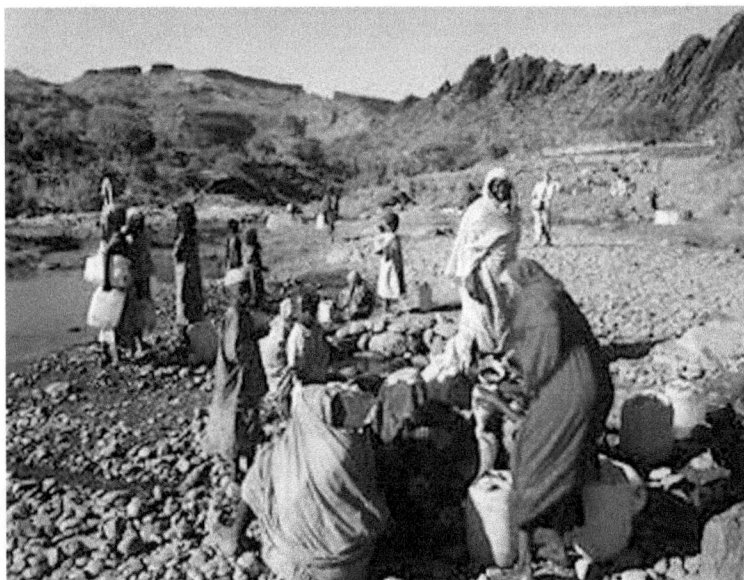

More excursion

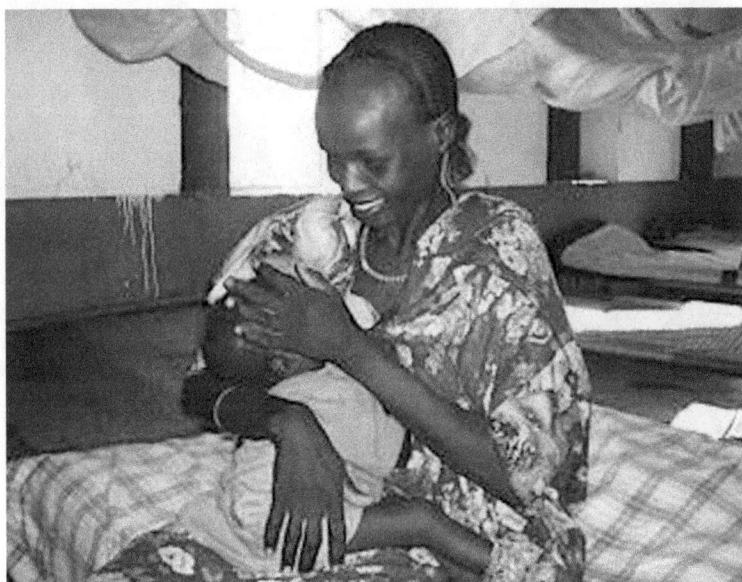

Inside pediatric ward, Golo

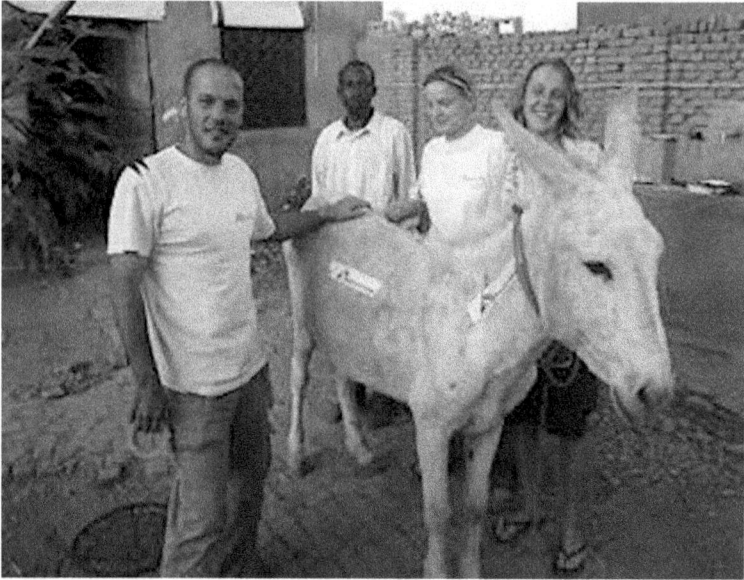

Jamal's donkey

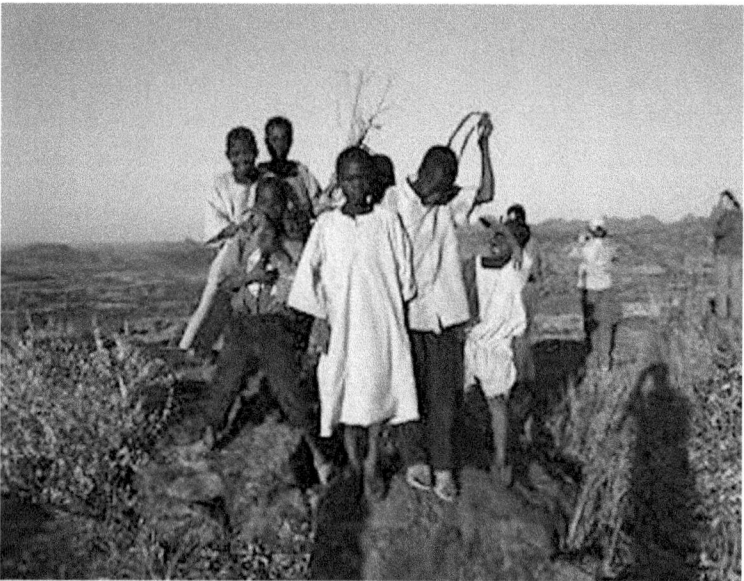

Sudanese boys

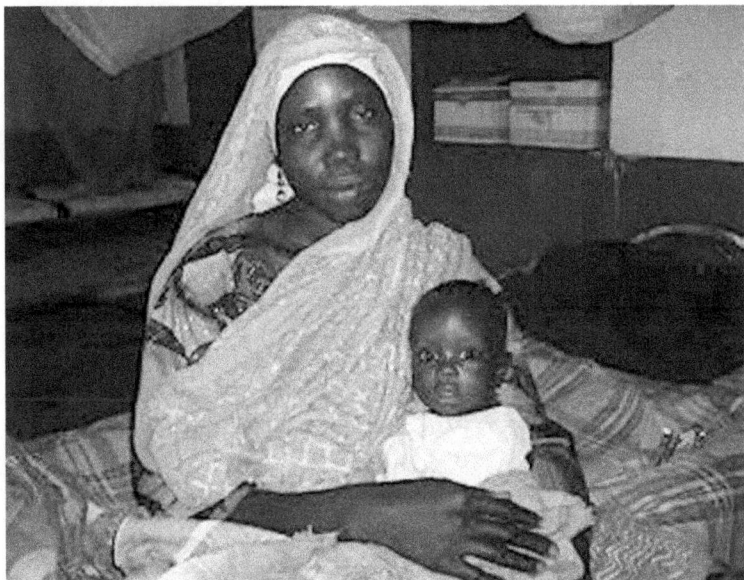

Child in Golo hospital, had been very ill

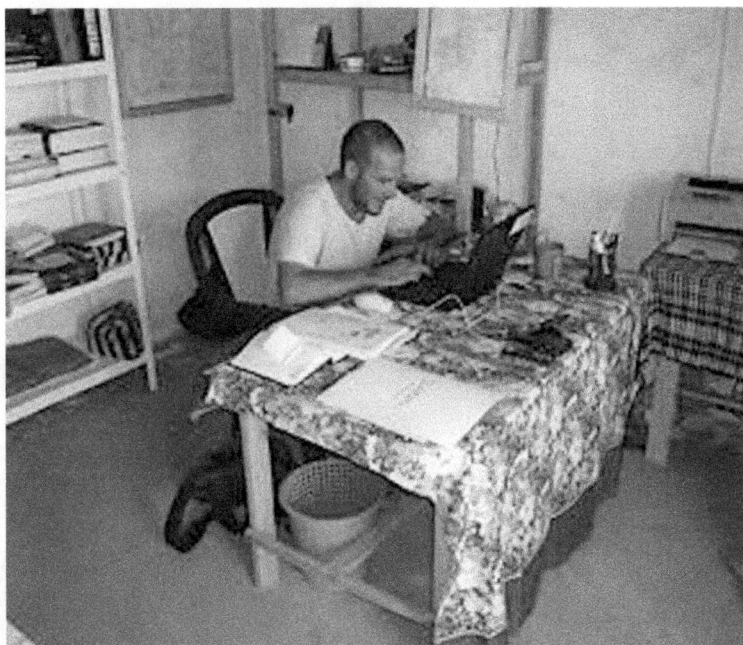

Damien in office in Golo

Therese's Dream

Dingila, Republique Democratique du Congo

Sent: Tuesday, November 10, 2009
Subject: One Day in Dingila, Republique Democratique du Congo

Hello, Bonjour, M'boti to All,

Well, I am not quite sure where to begin this story. Au premier, je veut remercier mes amis de Trois-Pistoles, Carol, Guylaine, Anne Marie, Camille, Emmanuel, et Patricia. J'ai eu besoin de toute la langue francaise que je comprends. I got on the bus in Portland, Maine, USA on the 1st of November, spent one night and one day in New York City, flew to Geneva via London, arriving on the afternoon of the 3rd (have rarely spoken a work of English since, except in Uganda), spent three days in Geneva, flew on the 6th to Entebbe, Uganda, spent one night in Kampala, flew on the 7th to Bunia, Congo (in a small plane seating about 12), spent two days there, then yesterday flew in a four-seat plane to Dingila, landing on a grass field. I have been in residence here for a bit over 24 hours.

For my friends from my trip to Sudan, it seems quite different here in many ways, similar in others. Traveling in the DRC (Democratic Republic of Congo) seems easier, less tension in the airports, less hassle with the officials, no one tried to charge me an import tax on my keyboard (yes, Darryl, I am still at it, and thanks Lynne, it made it in one piece and is working well). The land is much greener, very lush, dense trees as far one could see on the flight here. We are on a plateau at about 3000 feet, so it is not as hot as it could be, but quite humid, and it rained today, the first rain I have ever seen in Africa.

The people are almost as friendly as in Darfur, which is saying a lot. I am replacing a doctor from Cameroon, a very nice man who has tried hard to tell me as much as possible about the project here before he leaves in the morning. The field coordinator is from Sierra Leone, the logistician from France, there is a Congolese nurse, and me. C'est tout for now.

A Canadian nurse is expected in about a month. MSF is managing two small health centers, and trying to become more involved in the hospital. This will be one of my tasks, to work on developing a relationship with the local doctors in the hospital. My work will be much different from last year's, less direct patient care by comparison, more teaching and we hope collaborating with the local doctors. So far I have visited the hospital and the two health centers, met many people, been fairly successful at communicating in French, eaten much better food than was the case last year, and smiled and waved at about the same number of smiling people here as in Golo.

With the change in climate I have not seen the stars as in Golo, which will be a great loss if it continues.

There is a goodbye party for Dr. Narcisse which has just started here, and my presence is requested. I will try to send a weekly or so message. The security situation seems very calm at present, so I hope to not be reporting from any other part of the country for my 6 months here.

Hope all is well, bien, etc. in your part of the world.

Toujours, David

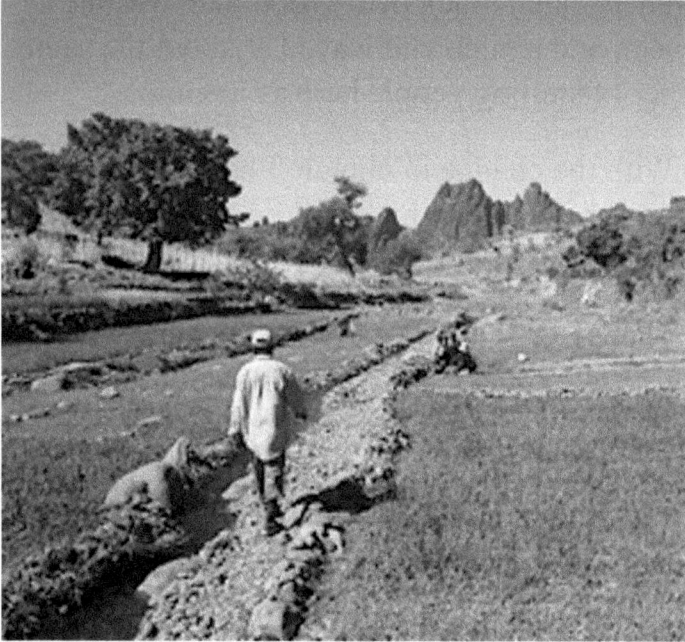

Mohammed Ibrahim leading excursion in Darfur

Sent: Sunday, November 15, 2009
Subject: Week's end in Dingila

Hello!

All continues to go well here for me. It has been raining hard for the past couple hours, lovely sound of rain on the roof. Quite a contrast to the five months in Sudan when not a drop of rain fell.

The other great meteorological contrast for me is the night sky. I have seen a couple of stars, generally the night sky is overcast, but what is lacking in brilliant stars is compensated with incredible electrical storms. Most every day there has been some activity, unlike anything I have experienced. The first storm began with flashes that I would call "heat lightening," lighting the night sky briefly, with little thunder. After perhaps an hour or so of this a traditional (for me) barrage of thunder and lightening (tonner et eclair) began, with extremely loud thunder, great flashes of lightening, and occasionally long bolts of lightening which advanced like slow moving shooting stars across the sky. The great lightening illuminated everything in the area. With the first storm there was little rain, but this morning it has poured. As the first storm subsided a few stars were visible, several varieties of fireflies flew by, and the lightening continued without thunder. Imagine, the whole show lasted for many hours! I finally had to give up and go to bed.

Living conditions here are also different. The house is fine, much like a western home but with brick floors. I miss my outdoor shower, which has been replaced by a plastic bucket in an old bathtub. I use a large plastic pitcher to apply the water to myself as I stand over the bucket in the tub. Leftover water in the tub is handy to flush the toilet. I would prefer the hole in the ground toilet of Golo to ours here with a broken seat, but it works fine. I have my own room, which recently gained an electric light thanks to our logistician, a nice youngster (25 years old) from France who grew up in Guateloupe, and has spent a fair amount of time in the US. We have a couple of good cooks, Gode during the week and Justin on the weekends, and the food is a big improvement over Golo, but for the vegetarians not the best. There is always some sort of local meat—goat, chicken, or beef—and we had a good fish from the Uele River, which flows through Dingila, a couple days ago.

There are rice, bananas generally, savory sauces for the entrees prepared by the cooks, a nice cake on one occasion, and often great orange juice (not from concentrate).

My main work here it seems will be to try to help improve the hospital. If one wanted to torture a western infection control committee member, this would be the place. Imagine a hospital without water, running or otherwise (no Purell either). We are planning to start next week if possible providing large containers of water and soap to the pediatric ward, plus providing some training with the staff. We will also be providing all the usual MSF medicines for pediatrics, with the goal of gradually extending our program to the other wards, which include maternity, general medicine, and surgery.

Up until now the local population has had to pay for health care and medications, which means many are unable to afford either. MSF is here at this time because there is a military group known as the Lord's Resistance Army (LRA) in the area, or at least close enough to cause whole villages to flee to Dingila for refuge. I will not try to recount the bizarre and tragic story of the LRA. Suffice to say that at this time it is a fragmented group of mercenaries who make a practice of terrorizing the locals, stealing food, goods, children, women, etc. A pretty unsavory bunch it would appear, who have succeeded in generating massive and well deserved fear. To emphasize, we are probably safer here in Dingila than in many other places, as there is a base of United Nations soldiers here, 17 in total. This may not seem like a large number, but the LRA presently consists of groups of 4 to 12 people who make occasional attacks with little in the way of weapons. Our job is to provide care for the displaced people and the locals.

In addition to the hospital there are three health centers which are quite busy treating many common problems: malaria, malnutrition in children, common infections, sexually transmitted infections, and a little bit of everything else. There is a psychologist who started the same time I did, also with MSF, a Congolese man named Andre. His mission is to work mainly with the victims of violence of all kinds, mainly with the displaced population, but also with the locals. It has been fun to spend time with him and learn his perspective on the world.

So far, knock wood, I have avoided the usual stomach upsets that accompany travel here, probably due to the excellent and extremely hot sauce I am adding to most of my food.

That is most of the story so far. I should add that I am speaking only French and this is going quite well, especially considering I have been here only one week.

For those of you who like to write to me here, it works best if you put my name (David is plenty) in the 'subject' box, and don't send pictures or any large attachments, as all the mail come through Geneva, and I guess too much volume is hard on the system!

So I need a brief update on the Boston sports teams, as I have been out of contact for two weeks. Thanks in advance!

Hoping that all is well with you all!!!!!

Love, David

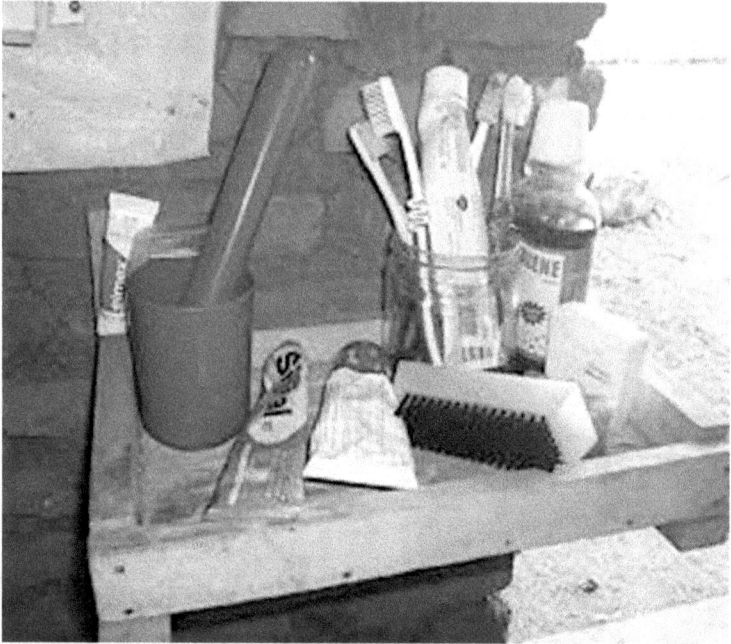

Communal bathroom in Golo

Sent: Monday, November 23, 2009
Subject: Dingila 3

Hello to All!

I will write a bit today (Saturday), then more tomorrow, I hope! This will be the first message sent under a new system. I will write to Carol, who will then send the news out to you all. The logistician here told me it is very expensive to send a large number of messages at once via the satellite system we use here, hence the new method. It is fine for you to write me directly using the address from my earlier messages, and again if you please write my name in the 'subject' place.

So, I am waiting for our regular cook to arrive to accompany her on her weekly trip to the market. Normally this would be a job for Nicholas, our logistician, but he is in Bunia this weekend for a little break, something I am told we are to have every six weeks. I am looking forward to the market experience.

We presently have a goat and sheep living in our yard, awaiting a party next week when they will be eaten, though the sheep escaped this morning. It remains to be seen if the guards can find him. The sheep may be lucky, as there are many animals wandering the streets of Dingila. Along with the two varieties mentioned above there are pigs, chickens, and some fairly big cows, who frequently leave their presents in the streets. There is a great crowd of birds nesting in a tree in our back yard, 20 or so nests. The birds are a pretty yellow color with dark wings, about finch size, with some orange markings around their faces. Their nests are the size and shape of softballs and hang from the branches. They are feeding babies now. I also, from time to time, see a pair of bright blue parakeets in a tree in our front yard, though lately they have been absent. Butterflies are a frequent sight, a firefly was in the bathroom last night, and some very large grubs can occasionally be seen crawling in the road.

We do our traveling of any distance on the back of small motorcycles driven by local drivers. It is nice to be traveling in the open air with a manmade breeze. I prefer it to traveling in the large Toyota land rovers that are one of the hallmarks of MSF. The small bikes are more in proportion to life here.

My work goes pretty well. We have had a very sick 10 month old girl in the hospital with malaria and possibly other infections. Three days ago it appeared very likely that she would die, but she has improved considerably since. Of course this is most rewarding, in a nutshell the reason to do this work. Another most interesting case involved preventing an intervention by the local doctors. A 33 year old woman was referred by one of our postes de sante (health centers) with abdominal pain, and the local doctors wanted to operate at once. Our Congolese nurse Omari and I saw the patient, and nothing seemed urgent. The conditions here are so profoundly unsanitary that surgery should always be the last choice. We treated her with antibiotics for what seemed most likely an infectious process, and she has improved. Ironically, after talking with her this morning it appears that she believes she needs an operation. The staff feel that they need to support the opinions of their doctors. The medical system here is profoundly, and to me disturbingly, hierarchical, of course with the doctors on high. Just another little challenge.

So now I have returned from the market, very lively as expected. We bought eggs (about $1.25 a dozen), four live chickens, oranges, shallots, sunflower seeds (I think), and some hot peppers to use in making pili-pili, a nice hot condiment which goes well with about anything. Needless to say I was quite the curiosity there. I did run into several people I had met before, which was nice, several who work for MSF here.

Last Sunday I went to the church of two of the local MSF staff here. They had invited me to attend, and were glad I did. The music was great, nice, rhythmical drumming by three guys while anywhere from five to maybe twenty people sang various songs, harmonizing. I was greeted as a special guest. This Sunday I have a date at the local Catholic church (the last one was protestant). There are many churches here, so I can probably visit a different one each week. And yes, there are many that look like the church from *Poisonwood Bible*, at least as it looked in my mind's eye.

Since I wrote the above we have been without internet access for two days. I want to send this off while I can! Hoping all is well with you all!!

Toujours, David

Hello Again!

It is interesting to me how quickly I become accustomed to the local environment and accepting of its 'normalcy.' The first few days feel like a documentary from National Geographic. The local houses are round and made of wood, mud, and thatched roofs.

Ours was built by the Belgians and looks quite European. But as time goes by the town and its people look natural. I guess it would be difficult to be somewhere for six months if it always appeared foreign, this quality of human adaptability probably has a lot of survival value.

The work in the pediatric ward of the hospital goes quite well. The very ill child I mentioned a while back recovered and went home, to the great joy of the parents and the doctor. We have been working closely with four local nurses who have been assigned to the pediatric ward, giving them some training on the MSF approach to medical care. So far they have been motivated and interested.

A Congolese medical student appeared a few days ago, at least that is when I learned of his student status. There are also many student nurses. The medical student has attached himself to me and wants to visit at out house this afternoon, hoping to learn something medical. I will certainly try to give him a hand with his studies. He seems to be a kind and gentle young man.

Three days a week, Mondays, Wednesdays, and Saturdays (today), I make rounds with the Congolese doctors, visiting all of the hospitalized patients. There are two Congolese doctors who share the rounding, one who just finished his training a few months ago, and one who has been here for three years. They are generally nice people, but their approach to both patients and nurses is foreign to me. I mentioned before the strict hierarchy they maintain. I have spoken some with the nurses about how different things are where I come from, and I guess they must see the difference. A couple of times I have questioned the medical decisions of the doctors (because they were obviously wrong), and everyone seemed quite surprised, and the doctors a bit defensive, but I think they are getting used to me, and it helps that I am old enough to be a father to all of them.

Unlike last year, I am not inspired to say much about the local physical environment. The exciting electrical storms have stopped for now, it is too overcast at night to see many stars, and the days become oppressively hot and humid by mid-afternoon, though thankfully it continues to cool down by nighttime. I occupy my free time with a little piano playing, listening to my music (mostly jazz masters, Darryl), and doing some reading. I am looking forward to the arrival of a Canadian nurse who should be here in a couple weeks. I like the people here, especially the Congolese nurse Omari who I work with every day, but the difficulties I have communicating complicated ideas in French gets in the way of deeper conversation, though for the purposes of daily life my French progresses well.

Hoping all is well in your corner of the world. Happy Eid today!!

Love, David

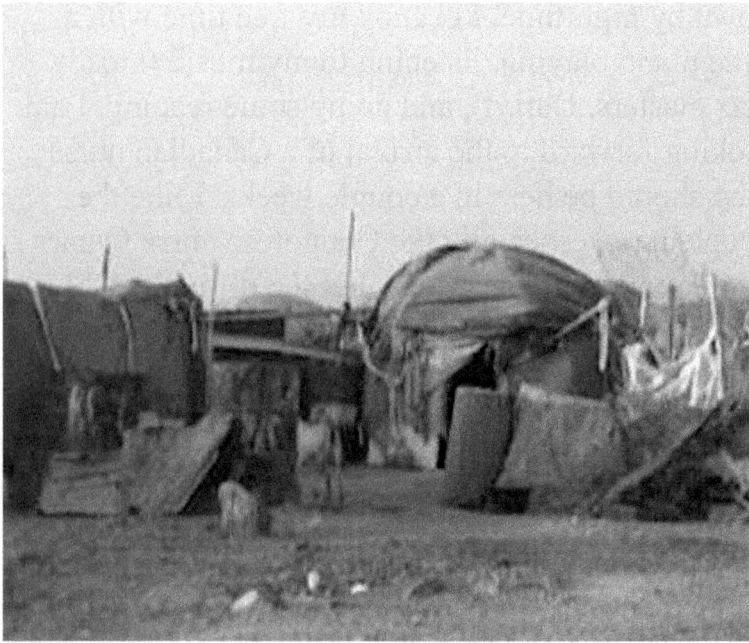

Slum in Djibouti

Sent: Friday, December 4, 2009
Subject: Dingila 5

Hello to all,

Quite an eventful week here, both good and bad as usual. Hard to believe only a week has passed since my last report. The time goes rapidly, while so much happens that it seems more time should have passed.

At this very moment I watch a large pig rooting around in our front yard, a pig about the size of Kelly and Anil's, if you happen to know them. My relationship with the animals has been interesting. One day walking home from the hospital I joined a mixed flock of sheep and goats, 20 or so, walking along with me, apparently unattended. Another morning, on the way to the hospital, I met a small herd of very large cattle with very large horns (will show you the pictures one day, I hope), and had to alter my route. Later that day the same flock of sheep and goats was grazing on the grounds of the hospital, perhaps the local version of the lawnmower. I have also been studying some very pretty lizards, multicolored with head one color, body another, and tail a third—orange, blue, and green, but I can't remember in which order. Quite a few pretty butterflies also, some like small Monarchs with distinct, colorful markings. Vultures fly over frequently.

Monday night we had a surprise visit from a group of United Nations soldiers, the group of Moroccans I mentioned earlier. One of them had been bitten on the foot by some aggressive ants (fomites) and suffered an impressive allergic reaction with swelling and pain in the foot and ankle and hives on much of his body. It was not a real emergency, as he had no trouble breathing, but he was miserable. The UN group has a nurse who had given him an injection of steroids (good idea), but apparently they had no other medications. Omari and I took good care of the young soldier, probably no older than 20 years. The group of four or five of them who came seemed very young (because they are), and really very gentle.

Hard to believe these children are holed up here ready to fight someone. They were very happy with our help (ibuprofen and antihistamines). The next morning I visited their base to check on the youngster and he was much better, smiling, and no longer limping. As I walked away from the base a passerby pointed out that someone was running towards me, and it turned out to be the commander of the soldiers, wanting to thank me. He was able to give a polite "thank you" in English, then we spoke a bit in French, all in all a lovely experience.

So now the hard part. The national staff had told me about a three-month old whose mother had died after a caesarian delivery. The custom here is to try to find a lactating woman to feed the child, and apparently someone tried to nurse the infant but was not very successful. But not a total failure either, as the child was still alive at three months. One of the local doctors asked if we had infant formula. We do not. We do have a therapeutic milk that is used for older malnourished children to slowly begin their re-feeding in the hospital. There appears to be no infant formula available in our community, which in most cases is a good thing, as clearly breastfeeding is the only reasonable choice most of the time (excepting the problem of HIV transmission and the case at hand). So finally this sad infant shows up at the hospital with the grandparents, who of course lost their daughter three months ago. The baby was very ill with fever, probable pneumonia, and though he did start drinking some of our milk, and of course did receive our good antibiotics, died about 12 hours later. Not much to add, the story speaks clearly for itself.

On the happy side, a most interesting medical case. The local doctors, who most of the time do not have access to any diagnostic testing, tend to give out the diagnosis of malaria to most everyone. We can test for malaria, so we felt quite smug when we could show that a child with fever and diarrhea, who was admitted with the malaria diagnosis, probably had only viral gastroenteritis. He really looked quite well at first, drinking well, but he became progressively worse over a couple days, and our smugness changed quickly to alarm when he lost consciousness and appeared, in the absence of laboratory studies, septic (severe bacterial infection). So we go from an apparently innocent viral infection to life-threatening illness, which fortunately we treated effectively with intravenous fluids and antibiotics (Ceftriaxone and Gentamicin), along with oral metronidazole when possible, presuming sepsis from the gastrointestinal tract). So this baby of eight months did well and went home after about three days of our intensive care!

So the usual balance of medical life in Africa continues, and this story will resume, I hope, next week! :)

Courage (as the French like to say here),

David

Sent: Saturday, December 12, 2009
Subject: Dingila 5

Hello Everyone!

As always a week of ups and downs. At this moment I would say that things are about even between the two, some children and adults doing well, some dying, but having received the best care we have to offer, so c'est la vie, ou la morte en cet cas.

The biggest positive for me has been the arrival on Tuesday of a Canadian nurse who (mes apologies a Trois-Pistoles!!) is an anglophone from the Yukon, originally from Toronto, who speaks French only a bit better than I do, ce que n'est pas trop mal au moment. I have truly enjoyed improving my French language skills, but it is like having a second job on top of the medical work, so by the end of the day my brain is thoroughly fried.

I had been looking forward to a break for a weekend in Bunia, where several Europeans speak english well. I may postpone the trip however, as since the arrival of my North American colleague it has been pleasant and relaxing to speak the mother tongue in the evenings.

For my friends at the Lovejoy Health Center, you will be pleased to know that the nurse's name is Trish. For those of you who don't know, I spent the past 10 years working happily with a nurse named Trish. At first I had been worried that the new Trish would not be comfortable with our living conditions in Dingila, but worry unfounded—she has been living in a tent in the Yukon without electricity or running water, works at a community health center with the Inuit Indians, and is a very lovely human being. So it has been fun, and a great relief, getting to know someone I will be working closely with for the next five months or so.

On the local medical front, there are major frustrations with the quality of care provided by the local system. We have essentially taken over the pediatric ward, and things generally go well there. We have introduced a formal charting system to record vital signs, note examinations findings, and to document the ordering and administration of medications. You probably would not believe the absolute disorder that reigns in the other wards, where orders are scribbled on little pieces of scrap paper, literally torn from notebooks that UNICEF provides for schoolchildren here. The scrap is given to the patient or their helper, who under the previous system (before MSF) would then go to the pharmacy to purchase the medications. Well surprise to me when the next morning the medication has not been given, or only half the dose, due to lack of money on the part of the patient. And why is the patient no better? There are other problems which the following case will illustrate.

A young man of about 25 years arrives with the diagnosis of myositis, a condition fairly common in the tropics, painful bacterial infection of muscle. The local docs are familiar with the problem and quickly made the diagnosis, but that is where the good news ends. These docs love any excuse to perform one of the simple surgeries they attempt here under unimaginably non-sterile conditions. In this case, during morning rounds, one of the docs stuck a hypodermic needle into the muscle in the back of the patient's upper leg, not a bad idea, to determine whether there was a collection of pus that would need to be drained. He removed the syringe which clearly had drained NOTHING, and announced that there was pus, and hence an operation was necessary. The procedure, making a large incision along the course of the hamstring muscle, was performed by the younger doc the next day, leaving the patient with a large surgical wound. At least the doc had the honesty to admit that no pus was found during the surgery. The young patient who had presented with a serious but not life threatening condition steadily deteriorated over the next several days. I learned the lesson described above, that medicines prescribed in morning rounds were by no means certain to arrive during the day. And it gets worse. We (MSF) are providing at no charge to patient or family all of the medicines used in pediatrics, and also often give medications to the hospital for general use, with the understanding that they are free to the patients. I personally, that is carrying them in my hands, gave a large supply of antibiotic (Cloxacillin) to one of the doctors for use in the hospital, and on morning rounds we discussed the fact that they would be available to the young patient with myositis, the proper dose being two vials given four times daily, and on we go. Two days pass and the patient deteriorates.

When I look at the chart it is apparent that he has received a total of SIX vials only over the course of three days. He should have received 24 vials. When the nurses told me the patient did not have the money to buy his medicine I lost it (for the first but not last time), gave a brief oration in my agitated French, marched to the pharmacy, grabbed enough medication for the next two days, and left them with the patient. Okay??

Two days later the patient is better, eating some, so far so good. Several days pass and the decline begins again. Why? He received the proper dose for two days, and though the order was to continue this medicine, no one took the 50 steps to the pharmacy to get more. I really lose it this time, but instead of ranting I do something intelligent. I implore my dear friend Omari, Congolese nurse working with and for MSF, to intervene. I did not witness the event, but

Omari tells me that he asked the nurses if they did not have a conscience, how could they let this happen, and having seen him in action on other occasions I am sure his message was stronger and more effective than one from me could have been.

So good, the medicine is restarted, but this time no improvement and in fact it appears that the patient will die. I am despondent, and have practically given up, when Trish arrives. She sees the man and wonders about the wound on his leg. I tell her the story and, voila, she starts thinking and talking about other sources of infection, like the fact that for much of the day this wound is soaking in the young man's excrement. So yesterday morning, in a sort of last resort mode, we add an injection of another antibiotic (gentamycin) and what do you know, the man is a bit better and taking liquids in the afternoon. It is early Friday morning, and I will not send this off for another day, so stay tuned.

One more story. A baby was born very prematurely, I would guess 32 or so weeks, 1300 grams, certainly the kiss of death here, and the baby did die. The birthday may have been the day Trish arrived. In any case, we were asked to look at the baby at the age of three hours. At this time, the baby had received, per order of the local docs, an injection of an antibiotic (ampicillin, not a bad idea, though neither mother nor child showed signs of infection) and two different steroid injections (hydrocortisone and dexamethasone, why either I have no idea). Aside from infection and hypothermia, the primary problem for the baby was going to be nutrition, as the mother's milk would not be arriving for a couple days. I was scratching my head about possibly using a feeding tube, which we have. There are no bottles for babies here. Trish suggested taping the tube to the mother's breast and encouraging the baby to suckle while sending the therapeutic milk we have down the tube.

Well, while I was struggling with something else, she arranged the feeding attempt, which took awhile (fetch some water, boil it, mix the milk, arrange the apparatus). After a bit I went over to check on how things were going. I stuck my head in the ward and there was a large group of nurses, mothers, family members watching as this tiny baby nursed away and finished the 20 ml of milk we had prepared. It may be difficult for you to understand what a truly wonderful and moving sight this was and continues to be for me, understanding that the baby died around the age of 12 hours.

Saturday morning, all the children in pediatrics are doing well, the guy with myositis looks a bit better but not yet out of the woods (or here it should be jungle), so they say. Wish them all well!

Courage, David

Sent: Friday, December 18, 2009
Subject: Dingila 6

Chers Amis,

Well, it has been quite a week for me, mainly for personal reasons. Last Sunday five of us took a lovely trip to the Bamukandi River, about 30 minutes from our house by motorcycle. The goal was a little break from the routine of our life here. After a sometimes bumpy ride we arrived at a large old bridge built by the Belgians about 50 or 60 years ago. It spanned a river probably 100 meters wide. A slow but steady parade of pedestrians and bicyclists crossed, most with goods heading to or from some destination.

We watched as a pirogue (fairly large boat carved from the trunk of a tree) left from one side of the river to ferry a person across, I believe providing a taxi service. The area along the river is quite dense jungle, cool that day in shade, pleasant contrast to the heat in the sun. Later we walked a ways down a trail that led to the launching pad of the pirogue, where five boats rested, ready for use, with a couple of paddlers available for duty. This being the end of my 5th week here, the excursion really served as a pleasant holiday of sorts, and reflecting on it now, just five days later, in the context of the past week, gives my mind a most pleasant repose. On the ride home I bought a couple bunches of bananas from a woman on the roadside, a tasty ending to a most pleasing day.

Then the trouble began for me. Each Monday I take a pill which is supposed to prevent malaria, though for me it has not worked very well, as once last year and again a few weeks ago I experienced this rather unpleasant illness. I have told myself, and it probably holds true, that my cases of malaria have been relatively mild thanks to this preventive medication, mefloquin or Lariam for those interested. This medicine is famous for certain psychiatric side effects.

I first took Lariam many years ago for a trip to India, and during my time in Sudan took the medication for five months without obvious problem. After taking it for about two months this year the fun began. My last weekly dose was four days ago. Over the past week my sleep had gotten progressively worse than usual, no trouble falling asleep but waking after about two hours with my mind just racing along, thinking about most anything, patients in the hospital, people I work with, or problems in the world in general. After a couple hours I would fall asleep for an hour or two, then up for the day. Needless to say, it was getting a bit tiring. I thought my problem was due to the background stress that is always present here, but I had never had a sleep problem quite like this in my life. Three days ago I went to bed at 9:00 pm, woke at 11:00 pm, and was up to stay. Something had to give. I also had a vivid nightmare (couchmare) in which the LRA were to kill me with poison gas. I really was not too scared by the dream, but it helped lead me to the proper diagnosis. Nightmares are one of the most discussed side effects of mefloquin, so when I read the detailed list of possible side effects—insomnia, agitation, tremor, tinnitus, nightmares, and several others—I was quite certain of the cause of my distress. So I am off the pill for now, and last night had a decent sleep.

We had a party last night for Nicholas who leaves today, having finished his tour here. It was a lot of fun. The locals get big time entertainment value out of watching me dance. I have also been working on my language studies in Lingala. One of the nurses in the hospital has made me a dictionary of common words (French-Lingala of course), and through talking with the guards and other local workers I have a vocabulary of about 10 to 15 words. I religiously greet everyone on the street on my walks to and from the hospital, including many small children who chuckle over my beginner's Lingala. This morning I was walking past two boys who had to be brothers, each wearing the same shirt, each with a piece of wood balanced on their heads. I could not resist taking the wood off one of their heads (it was a rather small piece) and balancing it on mine. They laughed, I did pretty well carrying it, and everyone was pretty happy for a moment. Yesterday I saw three tiny children walking hand in hand, side by side, aligned in order of height, the smallest coming up to my knee, and the other two an inch or two taller. If I had had my camera, the picture would be cover material for many magazines.

Trish left today on a six hour motorcycle ride as part of the vaccination campaign we have started. She will be gone for four days, back for a couple, then off again for a couple, then back to stay, inshallah. The caravan of motorcycles was pretty impressive, one bike with about 10 plastic chairs nested one on the other and tied down, two with large freezer boxes full of vaccines and ice packs, and other bikes carrying all materials necessary for a group of about 10 to live in the bush for several days. I took many pictures.

Omari left today for a three week vacation, having been away from his wife and three young children for five months. So as one might guess, with Trish and Omari gone, a child arrives with severe malaria and a hemoglobin of 4, very severe anemia, two years old, desperately needing blood transfusion.

On the bright side, just yesterday Trish and I prepared a kit with all the materials necessary to give a transfusion. The procedure generally requires much rigamarole, typing the child's blood, finding potential donors, usually family members, typing their blood to find a match, testing the blood of any potential donor for dangerous infections, then finally, if a match is found, drawing the blood and infusing it into the patient.

When we gave transfusions in Sudan we had about five people working for several hours to complete one transfusion, so my first thought was how can I do this alone. Well, I happen to know that my blood type is O negative, which means I can give my blood to anyone without causing them a problem, so end of story. The child needed only six ounces of blood, so no big loss for me.

Yesterday I was thinking what a fabulous thing it is to be here and to be able to help people, hard to describe the feeling, like trying to explain to someone who does not have children the feeling of becoming a parent. A truly heavenly experience, I commend it to you all.

So my friend with the myositis is still alive and possibly going to make it, all the kids are doing well in the hospital. Regarding transfusions, when we first arrived we lacked the materials to perform them, and suffered the miserable experience of watching two young children die, so you can see I was primed and ready to go when this child appeared today.

Hoping all goes well in Canada (east and west), U.S. (Maine to California), Holland, Switzerland,

and wherever else you good people may be at the moment!!

Love, David

Hello All!!

Hot, humid, and sunny, the weather report from near the equator at 1000 meters above sea level. Thankfully, it continues to cool down at night, so when the anti-malarial medicine finally leaves my body I may be able to start sleeping again. Feeling a bit better overall, but lack of sleep takes its toll.

The kids in the hospital are all doing very well. The 10 beds have been full most of the time, and we recently had our first case of severe malnutrition requiring hospitalization. Trish worked in a nutrition program with MSF last year, so she has been doing a lot of teaching with the local nurses, as have I.

The malnourished child comes from Bambessa,

a three hour motorcycle ride from here. Trish saw the child while giving vaccinations in the field and arranged for his travel to our hospital. She had called ahead so I prepared for his arrival.

We use a very formal protocol treating the severely malnourished, starting with a relatively low protein milk. When mother and child arrived they had not eaten. The child had been eating only rice for some time, causing his malnutrition. He is two years old. I brought food to the hospital for the mother, and technically should not have given any to the child, but that plan was not to be as the nutritional milk was not ready, so the child enjoyed a meal of fish, beans, and rice (the same meal we had just eaten) before converting to the nutritional milk, which he refused at first, but has been drinking happily since.

One of my own children had a birthday yesterday, and tomorrow is Christmas, so some differences between "our" and "their" experience. Congolese celebrate holidays with food. No presents. But thinking about my children reminds me of the greatest similarity between "our" and "their" experience. Parents here love their children deeply, and though they frequently experience the death of a child their loss is not less than ours, only less unexpected.

I received the sweetest gift today. Tired and a bit dazed by lack of sleep I made the rounds in pediatrics. The parents all greet me in Lingala, and I converse with them as best I can. While bending under the mosquito net of a tiny child's bed, reading her chart, this beautifully smiling girl looked me in the eye and said m'boti (hello) in the most straightforward and friendly fashion. High point of the day.

I may have mentioned we have a program for victims of sexual violence. There really is not a lot in this part of the country, far from the LRA atrocities. I would estimate that for the size of the community the rate of violence toward women is less than that of a large US city, probably similar to Portland, Maine, probably lower than Paris, France. Today I tended to a 14 year old girl who appeared much younger (11 or 12 years), who reportedly had been raped several months ago. The concept of this child's rape hurt, but the reality of this child's being inspired. She had told her story to the lovely Congolese woman Therese who is here to work with these women, employed by MSF. I got the medicines for the child to prevent or treat sexually transmitted diseases. Then I walked with Therese and this sweet child back to our house where we have vaccinations to give her for tetanus and hepatitis B. So walking and thinking about her I cry, while she smiles and engages us.

We reach home and the child has not eaten, it is noon. I serve her yesterdays leftovers and yes, a Coke from out "special" stock. So she is all smiles, gets her shots, walks back to the hospital with us, and on the way back happily tells Therese that this is the second time in her life that she has eaten mondele (white person) food. Tell me what this all means, I do not know.

Merry Everything a tout le monde!

Love, Papa David

Bonjour a tout le monde,

Quite an eventful week to report and it is only Monday! Thursday I will leave for a break in Bunia, returning the following Tuesday. The routine here is supposed to be a break of some sort every six weeks (I will have been here eight), first a weekend, then after 3 months a week of real vacation, then down the home stretch. I have started sleeping better, so hope to recover some energy during the break.

Last week the five month old son of one of our guards, Hadj, returned to the hospital for the third, and sadly final time in his young life. At two months he had pneumonia, before we arrived, and reportedly never recovered fully, returning a couple weeks ago with recurrent pneumonia, this time under our care. He seemed to improve well, but looking back on it the child was probably chronically malnourished, due to his ongoing illness. So 1 week after we discharged him he returned very ill.

All babies here exist in a precarious state for the first many months of life, I would guess that the mortality rate for all comers for the first year is horrifying, one can probably find it online if interested, and if you do let me know. So this very dear child was septic, severely anemic with a hemoglobin of 4.3, and never really responded to what we have to offer, including reasonable antibiotics and another transfusion (so one for two, running score). I was sitting with the extended family when the child died. Much wailing and tears, only tears from me. So the next day is the funeral which I attend.

We meet at the parents' home, 60 or 70 people arrive. After a communal song in the local language, a hymn I assume, the parents ride on a motorcycle with a driver, Hadj holding his dead baby wrapped in a blanket, his wife sitting behind him. The rest of us walk the mile or so to the cemetery, the motorcycle moving slowly and stopping from time to time to allow the pedestrians to catch up. I walk behind a woman I assume to be an aunt of the baby. Women walk on either side of her, arms interlocked. Several children, siblings I believe, cry and wail softly during the walk. It is Sunday afternoon with many people out and about. They all watch in respectful silence as the procession passes, and for the first time here I walk a distance without once hearing the cry of "mondele"— what a relief!

As we approach the grave site I notice several fresh graves. People must generally die at home, as not that many die in the hospital. Following the woman with her supporters I see their usefulness when, at the sight of the grave, she collapses, guided slowly to the earth by her friends. The family gathers around the grave.

First several of the baby's possessions are placed in the hole which is about four feet deep. A man, probably an uncle, stands in the grave and spreads the things around. Then he is given what appears to be a new piece of fabric which he opens, then the baby is passed to him, probably by an aunt, as both parents sob, Hadj looking away from the grave. The child is dressed in a pretty, simple white robe. He is wrapped in the new cloth, a layer of bamboo is placed over the baby and a heavy blanket placed over the bamboo, I assume to protect the baby from the earth. A woman who I happen to know, a nurse at one of the health centers we run, says a prayer, then another man, likely another uncle, begins shoveling the earth into the grave, while the man who was in the grave removes any roots or other debris from the dirt. Hadj and his wife leave as the earth fills the grave, and the rest of us follow.

It was good for me to get back to the hospital later that day, to return to the routine of work. All the other children in hospital are doing well at the moment. Today, the day after the funeral, people seem to greet me in a more friendly way, not that they had been unfriendly before.

Other stories I had in mind to report were trumped by this, so will close for now, there may be another report before I leave for the weekend.

And, for your information, I always like to hear news from home (yours) or comments or anything, so please do not hesitate to write, I am especially interested in reports from Amsterdam!

M'boti mingi (au revoir ou bonjour en Lingala),

David

Sent: Wednesday, December 30, 2009

Subject: Dingila 9—Therese's Dream

Hello,

The full moon is bright this morning and I am up early. I will fly to Bunia later today for the weekend break. I have a long list of things to get there for our staff. Many of the Congolese who work for MSF here are in their 40's, so reading glasses top the list. David wants Cokes and mayonnaise. Trish asks for carrots and whatever other vegetables are to be had there. Therese wants sugar which I assume must be of better quality than what we can buy in the market here.

The local businessman Prosper, who we visit many evenings for a beer or a Coke, asks for a soccer ball for his children. Not sure if Andre has put in an order yet. I am looking for some medical books to "borrow" from the crew in Bunia, hoping for an old tropical medicine textbook. Should be fun at the market there!

I will make a quick trip to the hospital this morning before leaving. Trish will hold down the fort (English expression for being in charge) while I am gone, we went to the hospital together last night to look over the patients. A three year old boy came in a couple days ago in a coma with severe malaria, pneumonia, and a hemoglobin of 3.6 (very severe anemia, the worst I have ever seen), and seems to be doing okay after a couple doses of the usual medicines and some blood. All in all things are going pretty well.

Therese is the lovely 31 year old Congolese woman who works with the women here who have experienced sexual violence. She also is the grandmother of a beautiful seven month old girl who at present is in the hospital with diarrhea, not too serious, and getting better.

I spent a soothing few minutes yesterday sitting in a chair in the office of Andre and Therese, just holding and playing with this child. Therese recently went to Bunia for some job related training, a very big deal for her as it was her first airplane trip, as certainly the overwhelming majority of Congolese will never fly in an airplane.

Several days ago, during the Monday morning meeting we have with the nurses who work for MSF, Therese says to me "I had a dream about you last night." So after everyone has a good laugh for the obvious reason, she recounts her dream. I am driving a land rover, the standard MSF vehicle, and Therese and her sister (who I do not know) are the passengers. The road is very rough and dangerous, with a river to the right and a drop off to the left. I am a good driver (in her dream, at least), and in this dream she knew that I was the chief of MSF doctors. Quite interesting, eh?

So, looking forward to a little break, the happiest of New Years to all of you, 10 years after the start of the Millennium (reminds me of a song!).

All the best, David

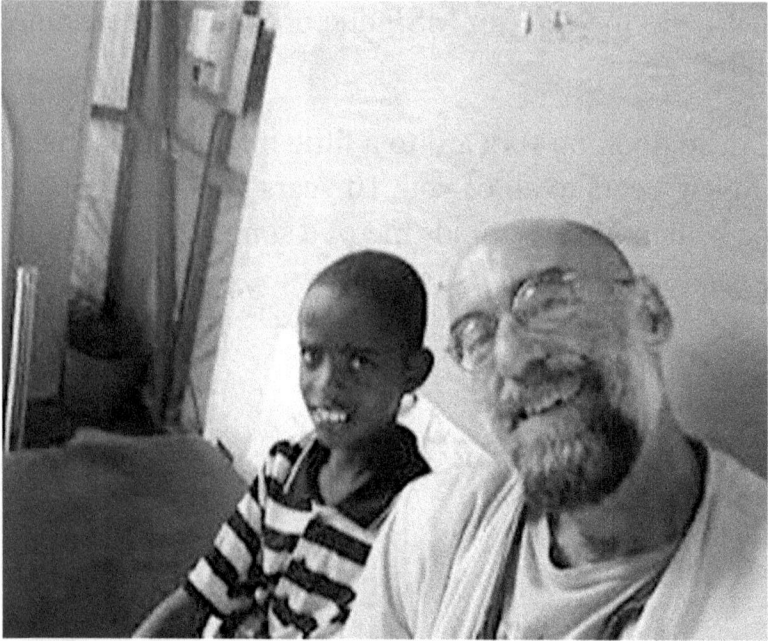

David and Friend

Hello a tout le monde,

Quite the remarkable coincidence occurred on my arrival in Bunia last week for my break. We were met at the airport by a Congolese man named Pierre, very friendly and helpful with the journey through customs. He works for MSF there, helping to coordinate flights. During the car ride from the airport he asks where I am from. United States. Which state? Maine. So he tells me that his brother and his family live in Portland, Maine, which is about 100 kilometers from my house. So now I have the brother's name and phone number, and a Congolese friend to visit on my return to Maine. Later that evening Pierre told me that he had already spoken with his brother about me. Small world?

New Year's Eve was spent at a place the United
Nations operates as a sort of restaurant/bar for their
staff, which is quite large in Bunia. Unlike Dingila
where we are the only westerners, Bunia is swarming
with NGO's (non-governmental organizations). It is a
much larger city than Dingila, maybe 20,000 people, a
couple restaurants, many small shops.

The highlight of the trip for me was shopping
for the Dingila team, both for our general food order
and the things people had requested. I was able to
find almost everything on "the list," so everyone
here has been quite happy with me. I went to a large
market with Abdullah, a Congolese logistics assistant
working with MSF in Bunia. He spent about seven
hours working with me on Saturday, supposed to be
his day off. I tried to buy him lunch at a restaurant, but
the best I could do was entice him to eat some leftover
food from one of the MSF houses.

We had a good time together I think, at least it
was good for me, and he laughed much of the time,
so I hope it was relatively pleasant for him. He helped
me buy a shirt for myself, and I gave him the one I
was wearing (not a great sacrifice, both shirts cost
about $6 US). As a generalization, the Congolese
people laugh a lot and laugh well, deep belly laughs.

There are some interesting cultural differences.
The day after the funeral I described earlier I saw the
nurse who had spoken a prayer at the graveside. When
I told her that I really liked her prayer she started
laughing heartily, in the presence of several others,

leaving me mystified until I questioned a Congolese coworker about it. He told me that often people laugh here when they are very happy about something, so my compliment made her happy, and even though it was in regard to a very sad situation, she was responding to her happiness.

I have been meaning for several "reports" to comment on the smell of human beings. Most people bathe regularly here, but no one, myself included, uses deodorant, and most work hard. People smell about the same in this situation. Perhaps a worthwhile screening test for westerners wanting to work here would involve assessing their level of tolerance for the smell of people without perfume. As a youngster I enjoyed the smell of the locker room, and have always been happy not to use deodorant. Trish told me yesterday that she could smell me from outside the house (she stays in a separate house next door). I had not yet taken my morning shower. The long and short of it is I like the way people smell here.

The work in the hospital goes well, only one child has died in the six weeks we have been running the show, and things are really quite busy, with most of our 20 beds full most days. A few days ago we gave another transfusion to a beautiful little girl of about eight years who appeared to be close to death, unconscious with a hemoglobin of five due to malaria. Her hemoglobin had dropped from seven to five over two days, not unusual with severe malaria in a child. She looked great last evening.

133

This afternoon Trish and I will give our first formal teaching session to the nurses and nursing students at the hospital. We are going to start with a discussion of malaria in its various clinical forms, from the MSF perspective, which is quite different from theirs. Should be interesting. We have been working closely with four or five of the nurses in the pediatric ward, so they should be converts to our point of view, as they have seen how well the kids are doing with our approach.

It has been great to hear from many of you, any news from your home always appreciated!!!! So a happy and prosperous New Year to all!!

Love, David

Hello!!

For the past week I have started a new morning ritual, yoga on the veranda before the sun rises. So far it's 12 sun salutes, some leg raises, a long shoulder stand, a few twisting poses, and a child to finish. Off and on over the years I have taken classes, most recently with Lillian, my favorite teacher. But, though I have always enjoyed the classes, this is the first time I have practiced on my own. Trish is a fantastic practitioner, and one session with her prompted my independent practice. There is not much opportunity for exercise here, very hot much of the day. We walk a lot, but the cool hours of the early morning are the best time for something more, and I actually

face the spot where the sun will rise. This morning
the noises from the dark included not only the ever
present sound of insects and some unidentifiable (to
me) animal noises, but also drumming in the distance,
followed a bit later by what seemed to be a drummed
response from elsewhere. Most interesting.

We had a remarkable day in the hospital
yesterday. A six month old girl arrives in terrible
condition, a malnourished stick figure weighing
5.6 kg, or 12 pounds, fever of 40 degrees (axillary,
very high), and a hemoglobin of 4.6 (another severe
anemia). Wow, one cannot be much sicker than
that in the living state. So after a dose of antibiotic
(ceftriaxone), an injection for malaria (artemether),
it was time for a transfusion. The amount of blood
given is based on the weight of the child, and less is
given to severely malnourished children for fear of
causing heart failure, so in this case the calculated
amount was 60 ml, which translates to two ounces or
four tablespoons of blood. Not much. So several hours
later the child is alert and drinking quite vigorously
the therapeutic milk we have to supplement
breastfeeding. I am writing early Tuesday morning,
and will update later, but at the moment there begins a
most beautiful African sunrise which I go to watch.

Now Wednesday morning, the sunrise was
great, may be another soon! So this is how the work
goes here. The children above do well yesterday,
but way too soon for the final verdict. This morning
I see a child who had been doing okay it seemed,
a four month old (always trouble, the younger the

worse) who came in with a fever, not much on examination, the Paracheck (one of our few useful tests, very reliable for the worst variety of malaria, but not useful for the other three) was negative, so we are treating for probable pneumonia, and initially the child improves, fever down over a couple of days. Yesterday morning a low grade fever returns, Paracheck again is negative, and the child appears pale. I wanted to check for anemia then, but our only machine was off at one of the health centers to be used to screen pregnant women, to return to us in the afternoon. I thought that would be soon enough, as the child did not really look terrible, and I had decided to treat her for malaria based on the clinical picture, even with the negative test.

We were taught in medical school to treat the patient and not "the numbers," numbers referring to the results of the innumerable tests we order routinely in the western world. The rule applies even where only one or two tests exist. So when we return to the hospital in the afternoon the child looks much worse and the heart examination was most remarkable, heart rate of 172 with the most distinctive gallop rhythm I have ever heard (for the non-medical, the normal heart sound includes two distinct sounds per beat, while this child's heart was producing three sounds of equal volume, something I had previously only heard in elderly patients with heart failure). It all made sense medically (only medically) when we learned that the child's hemoglobin was 2.7, the new record low. So this small infant received, I hope, (the transfusion was not complete when we left the hospital) five tablespoons of blood. Will report more later.

Thursday and not sleeping so well this morning. The tiny malnourished baby dies during the night. I am afraid we could have done some things differently that might have made a difference, but certainly not possible to know for sure. When there really are so few medical variables to monitor it is difficult to feel that something was neglected. Basically, looking over the chart the next day, this tiny child had lost a significant amount of weight overnight, and had continuous diarrhea according to his nurse, a lovely man named Jean. I had not noticed the loss of weight, perhaps too confident that the child was doing well after antibiotics and blood. Hard to acknowledge cause of death as dehydration. On the brighter side, the child with the record low hemoglobin looked much better yesterday, but not yet time for celebration. It seems to me that it is all too easy in a setting like this to take on the attitude that, when there is a bad medical outcome, it was unavoidable due to the difficult medical circumstances. Sometimes this is clearly true and sometimes not. However, it is practically certain that all the babies discussed above would have died if we had not been working here.

I simply think it is wrong for me to apply a different standard to my work, while acknowledging the limitations on what one can do here, than I would at home. I "lost it" a bit around this issue last night after dinner, these general ideas about my responsibility suddenly hitting me while the rest of the team was having a pleasant moment. I feel supported by the team here, but they probably think I am a bit crazy, and as many of you know they are probably right.

Thanks for listening!! Will keep you posted.

Love and Courage, David

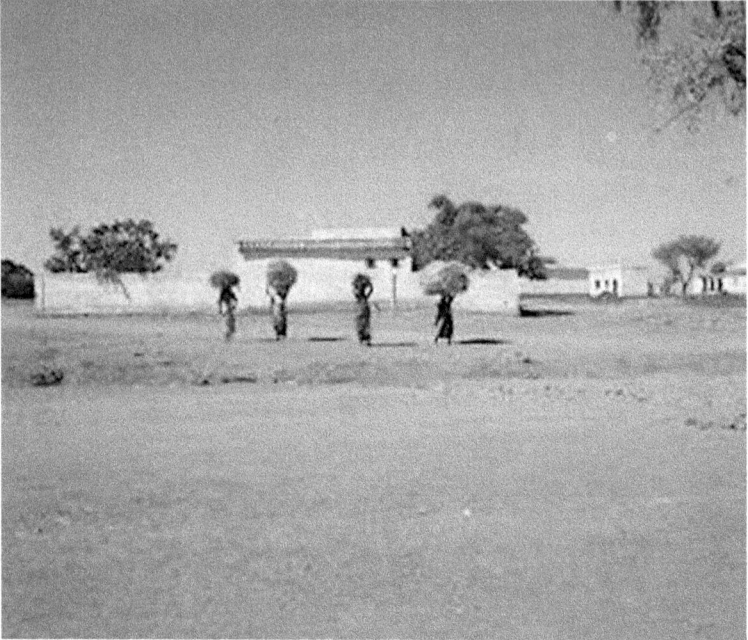

A typical village scene in Golo, Sudan

Sent: January 22, 2010
Subject: Au revoir a Dingila

Hi All,

Well, to my surprise and sadness I am heading home sooner than planned. Apparently the powers that be feel it is not wise for me to return to Dingila. From their point of view I can understand that they fear my behavior may have been more due to the stress of work than to the medication effect, so they fear a repeat performance if I return. From inside my head it is clear that this is not the case, but I have not been able to get the inside of my head into someone else's. So I leave for Kampala today, then on to Geneve sometime soon, then to New York, then on to Maine.

As always a silver lining, looking forward immensely to seeing family and friends, plan to visit Cristina in Geneve and Stuart in Geneve or Basel.

This morning I was walking to the hospital in Bunia to give them a little of my blood for the road, so to speak. I was a little down, but found myself walking along with 2 tiny Congolese girls, 5 or 6 years old, carrying backpacks almost as big as themselves, backpacks for school, not to carry wood from the forrest. They smiled broadly, chatted together, holding hands, running at times, such a lovely sight I could not help but feel hopeful for this sometimes too sad world.

Courage and Love, David

Second Intermission

The effects of the mefloquine (Lariam) were long lasting.

I continued in a manic state on my return, telling the folks in Geneva that I was fine and wanted to return to Dingila, then from the US insisting that my MSF New York friends arrange for me to go to Haiti ASAP to help after the massive earthquake.

They ultimately obliged and I spent four weeks there in an generally unrewarding position as a medical doctor in an orthopedic hospital. Most of our patients were young with only orthopedic problems, and with the older ones with other medical problems like diabetes, we often lacked necessary medications, like insulin. Another frustration was, ironically, an overabundance of Haitian doctors. With the destruction of hospitals and clinics by the quake many Haitian doctors were desperate for work. I felt that I was taking a spot that they should have occupied.

After a week or two in Haiti my manic symptoms faded, and were replaced by a deepening depression. Around this time I heard from my dear friend Ken Eisen that his wife Beth, also one of my closest friends, who had been diagnosed several months earlier with ovarian cancer, was not doing well.

I decided to return to Maine early (I was supposed to stay in Haiti eight weeks) and offer my time and energy to Beth and Ken. Helping care for Beth was very healing for me, and slowly my drug induced depression lifted.

After Beth died I returned to work as a country doctor, returning to my old practice in Maine. Two months after Beth died I moved into a spare room in Ken's house. We made quite the odd couple, both struggling to get on with our disrupted lives. We took a vacation together with two other friends, visiting Morocco, my first trip to Africa as a tourist. Several months later I was contacting MSF for another assignment, one which would turn out to be both my most difficult and most rewarding.

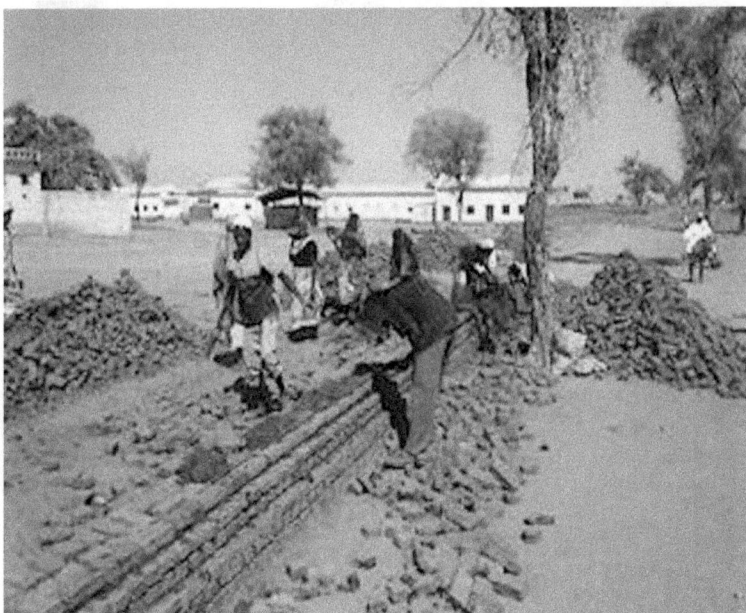

Community project, building a wall around Golo hospital

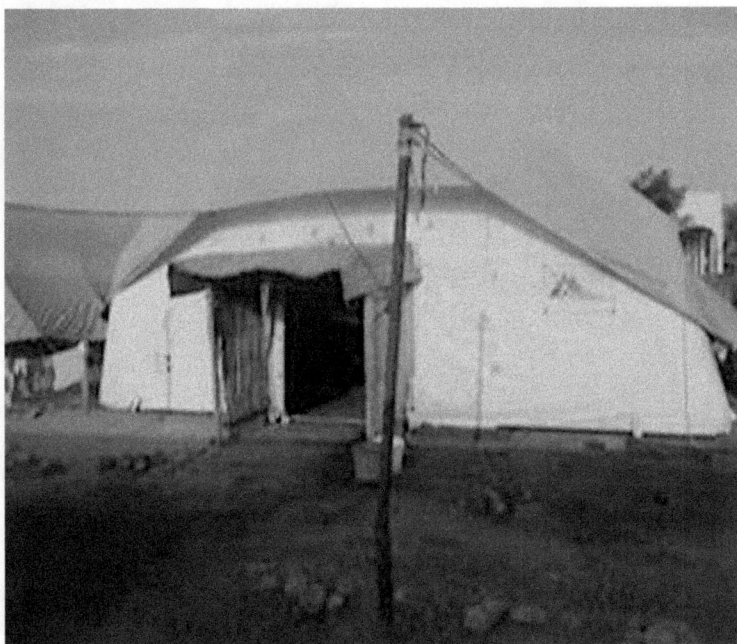

Tent hospital in Djibouti

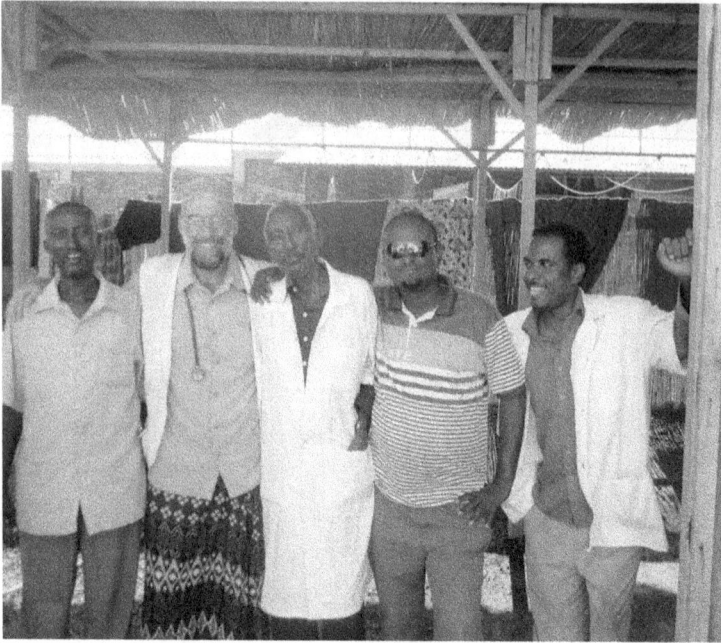

Group December 29, 2011

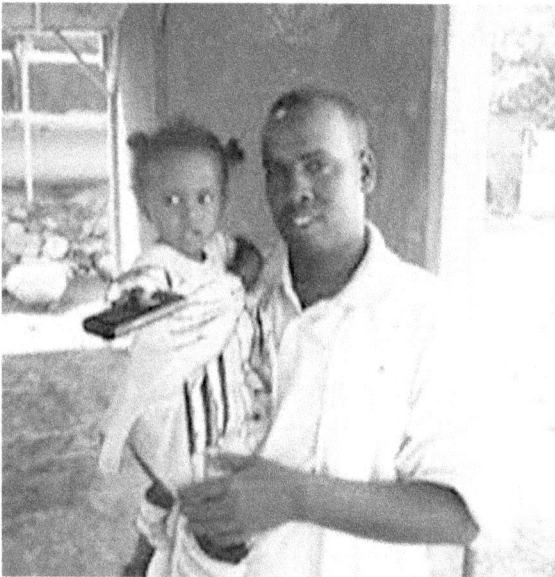

Superb nurse and child

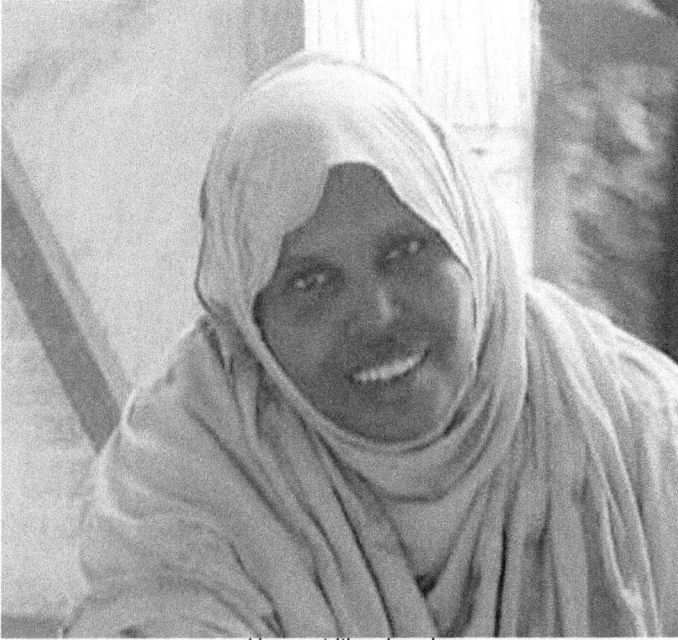

Uma nutritional worker

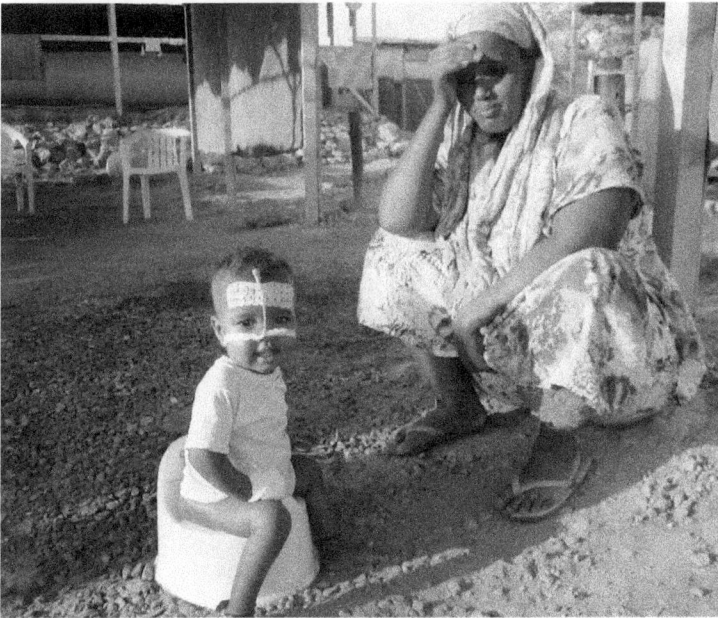

Recovering baby patient

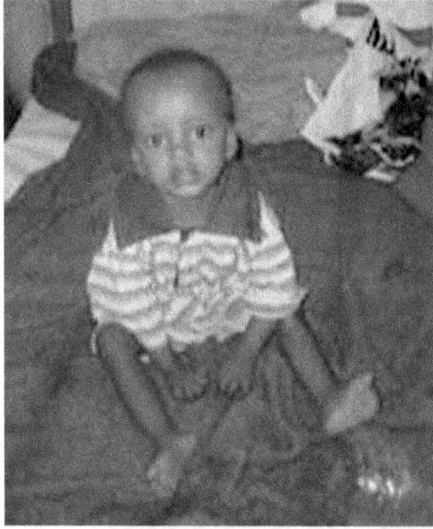

Child had been near death December 3, 2011

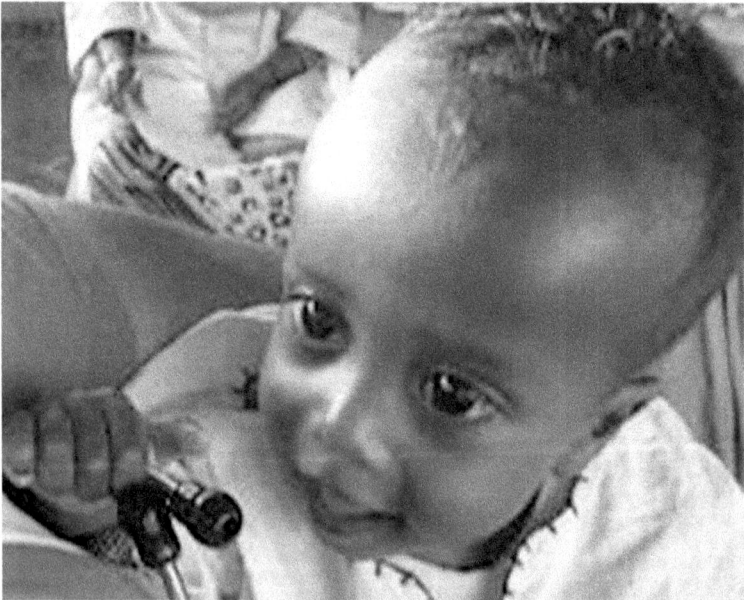

Sweet child

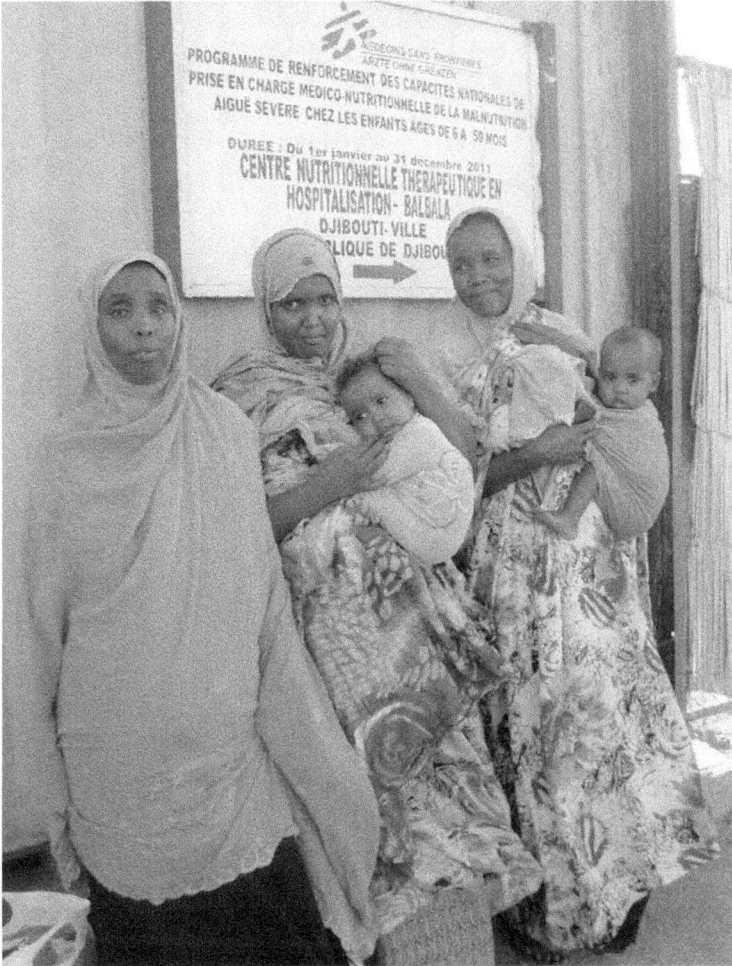

January 5, 2012

Djibouti

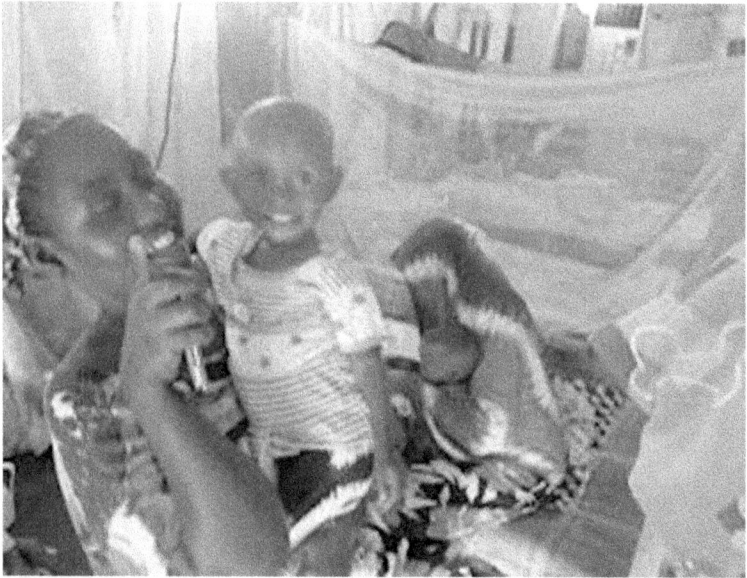
Happy customer

Hi!

After spending a week in Paris visiting a family
I met while traveling in Morocco, with the goal of
improving my French (which was accomplished,
at least to some extent, and as a bonus I got to see
Paris), after visiting my friend Stuart and his family
in Basel, Switzerland, and after spending less than 48
hours in Geneve (supposedly getting oriented for my
trip here, in reality having a great visit with Cristina,
Xavier, Hector, and Zinnia), I began a 20 hour airport
adventure, traveling from Geneva to Frankfort to
Addis Ababa to Djibouti. There is a direct flight a
couple of times a week from Paris to Djibouti, but
this was booked into November. So I have been here
for three days, getting oriented to the people I will be
working with, the place, and my future job.

I will be one of two doctors in charge of an inpatient program, a field hospital, for malnourished children with medical complications which require hospitalization. Such complications are commonly pneumonia and diarrhea, no malaria this time. The doctor I am replacing is a very competent woman from Italy, Dr. Emma, who trained in infectious diseases. She has been working with, and I will continue working with Dr. Alfonse, an African from Guinea, on the other side of the continent. The nurses in the hospital are all locals, most Djiboutians and some Ethiopians. Most are French speakers, the Ethiopians and others who trained in Ethiopia speak english well. The rest of the expat team includes a logistician from France, Jerome, very nice guy, a human resources woman from Tunisia, Nizet, also very friendly and helpful, and the head of the project here is a man from Mali, also a medical assistant, named Kali. He went on vacation the day after I arrived, so I haven't yet spent a lot of time with him, but he seem friendly and competent.

Yesterday I met with the expats here and spent a chunk of time with Emma at the hospital, which is called the CNTH (centre nutritionelle therapeutique). There is room for up to 60 children, ages six months to five years, and there are around 50 patients at present. Some of the recent arrivals are really quite sick, most who have been here awhile are doing pretty well at the moment. I have done some of this work in Sudan and Congo, but never in such a large program. Should keep me busy, and again it is comforting to not have to dive in and flounder my first day here!

My life here will be quite different from my past two African experiences. Djiboutiville, where I am living, is a city of about 400,000 people. The hospital is located in the middle of a miserable slum, while the house I live in is quite opulent. The folks in Geneva explained that there is really nothing in between as far as living goes. The city has both French and American military bases. The country is a former French colony, and in the present world holds a strategic location for US "interests." Much money flows into the country to develop the harbor, global money which as usual spreads only a few crumbs to the local poor. A lot of work for the prostitutes in the downtown bars. The local people have been friendly, not at all surprised to see white skinned people. All the mothers in the hospital dress in lovely african colors, as in Sudan. Almost all are Muslim.

My head is full of French all the time which is good for me, but I will admit I was happy to learn that the logistician who will arrive in a couple days to replace Jerome is from Australia. It is always nice to be able to speak with an anglophone, especially when tired in the evening.

So I am getting hustled out of the office, so will close for now. I have modern internet access here so you can write me directly and I can keep track of my Boston sports teams without special help.

A toute a l'heure, David

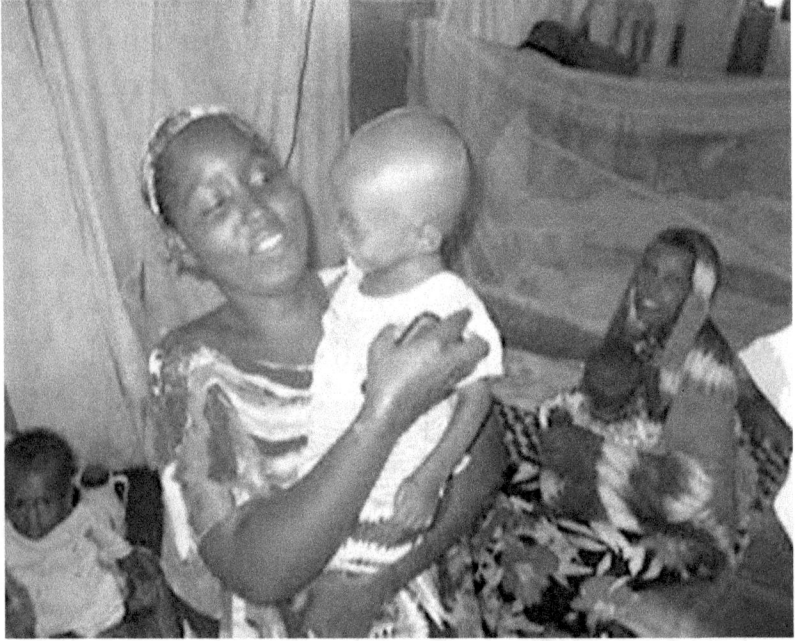

In hospital

Sent: Friday, October 28, 2011
Subject: Djibouti 2

Bonjour! Nabad! (Somali) Mahise! (Afar)

Another sunny day in Djibouti. Did I already say it is pretty warm here, very dry, not too much greenery. The colorful clothing makes up for the lack of flowers.

For most of the week I shared the work with Dr. Emma. Great fun working with her. She is a good role model for working in a stressful setting with many distractions, always composed and with bountiful patience. Next week I will start sharing the night call, which promises to be challenging. Most of it is by phone, and the challenge will be to understand what is being reported in second language French or English. Some of the nurses who will be making these calls are very good, and some are not. Emma knows who to believe and who to question, and has passed a lot of that on to me, but I have yet to learn half of the people's names (of the 50 or so I have met), so in reality I will probably not know who I am talking with. It is a bit of a hassle actually going to the CNTH (hospital) to see the kids at night, involving calling a driver , then about 15 minutes of driving to get there. Emma says many of the calls at night are not serious, but it is often hard to tell, so I will probably be traveling a bit before I feel comfortable working by phone. Alfonse, the African Doc, practically never goes in at night, a function mainly of experience but to some extent also personal preference.

I have seen some remarkably sick children over the past week, all of whom have gotten better. They arrive in a state of chronic malnutrition, and on top of this some serious infection, so far mainly gastroenteritis or pneumonia. Several were in shock when they arrived, essentially unconscious and barely responding to the placement of intravenous lines. The nurses here do pretty well at starting these lines, good thing they don't have to rely on me for this! All of these very ill children are given intravenous fluids, then antibiotics, as we have no reliable way to tell whether their infections are caused by bacteria or viruses. So for this week at least, these children who arrived on death's door all did well, some up and walking the next day, a truly remarkable thing to witness. Most of the admissions to the program are not that acutely ill. They suffer chronic malnutrition

which becomes complicated by an infection
which leaves them unable to maintain even their
malnourished state.

These children may require only rehydration
by mouth or if needed by a tube placed via the nose
into the stomach, and removed once they are eating
normally. Feeding is started with specially formulated
therapeutic milk, then a high calorie paste is added
when they are able to eat it. The paste is pretty tasty,
so most kids eat it eagerly. Their time in the hospital
ranges from less than one week up to six weeks in
exceptional cases, most stay between one and two
weeks. We discharged nine children yesterday so
the census now is around 50, as five new cases were
admitted the same day.

Tuberculosis is quite common here, some of the
kids come into the hospital already under treatment.
If a child is not gaining weight after treatment for
two weeks, we send them to a tuberculosis center for
evaluation, which includes chest x-ray and treatment
for TB if indicated. One child who had been in the
program since before I arrived died during the week,
the first death in about a month, which speaks very
well for the program. This child was a two year
old who weighed slightly less than nine pounds (4
kg). Imagine that. The child had been in and out of
our program several times during his brief life. He
almost certainly had some sort of serious underlying
condition. Dr. Emma was quite attached to the child,
having seen him through a couple of hospital stays.
When I first met him I could not believe he was living,

hence I was not at all surprised to hear he had died, but I certainly can understand Emma's response. Not too much time for tears here, as the next sick one is on the way, and in any case the program is impressive, and most kids are doing very well.

Last Saturday I played in a soccer game, the medical staff against the logistics staff. Jerome and I were the only white faces in the game, I am quite sure I am 20 years older than the second oldest, and here is the big news for the week, I scored the only goal for our team!! We lost 2-1, but as my teammates pointed out the goal was a face-saver for us. It was really quite funny, the next day several of the national staff mentioned the goal. I am not about to consider a career change, but playing was fun. There may be another game tomorrow.

Brian, the Australian logistician replacing Jerome, has been here for a few days. He is very nice, a 25 year old already on his third mission with MSF. Great for me now to be able to speak with a native English speaker. His French is better than mine, largely because he spent 6 months in Quebec Province as a 16 year old high school student. He was in a rural community where only French was spoken, about half way between Montreal and Quebec city. Last night was the start of our weekend in this muslim country, and everyone likes to go out to the disco. I went with the group and had a remarkable experience. While dancing with Brian (most people were dancing in same sexed groups), a man approached me saying he thought he knew me. And indeed he did!! He was working for MSF in Bunia, Congo during the time I was in Dingila, and we had spent a bit of time together when I passed through Bunia. He now works for another organization, Action Contra Faim (ACF), a French organization working to provide nutritional support. This group actually took over the outpatient nutrition programs that MSF was running in Djibouti. Proponents of the "small world" theory take heart.

So when I am not working, scoring goals, or disco-hopping I am playing my keyboard a good deal (thanks again, Lynne) and reading quite a bit. Brian says he likes to cook, and since we are on our own on Fridays we may do some cooking this weekend. Again it is so far, so good from here. I am sure it will be more stressful when I am working at night on my own. The on call duties will be split between myself and Dr. Alfonse, so there should be enough time to catch up!!

So I sign off for now. Hope you all have a good weekend!

A la prochaine, David

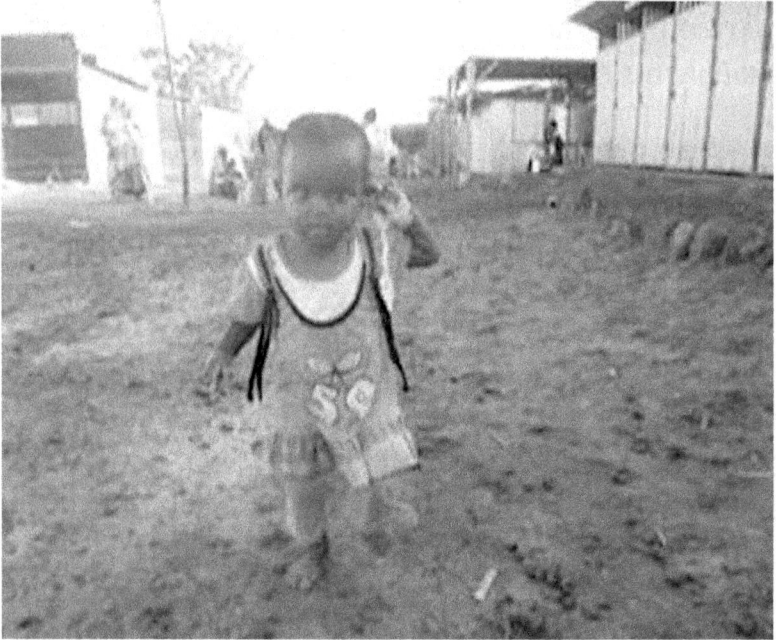

Little patient friend

Sent: November 11, 2011
Subject: Djibouti 3

Hi All,

Things continue to go well here. I am on call this weekend, which started last night. Will describe call so far in a second, but on my way to the office I ran into a young man from Washington state who works for the US Embassy here. We had a nice chat, the first American I have seen in three weeks. He says there are only a handful of Americans outside of the military who live in Djibouti, one who runs a restaurant, a couple who work for NGO's, and an oddball or two. So an interesting side bar to the day, will probably get together with him and his buddies. He already invited me to the grand opening of the new embassy building, the biggest building in Djibouti (again, no comment), in December. I might even go!

So back to life here, I have been on call at night

three times. The first night I was quite nervous, slept little, and got one phone call that amounted to nothing. The second night I was sleeping well when the call came in that an infant was very ill, I spent two hours at the hospital, the baby survived for a few days but never really regained consciousness, and died this morning. Last night I would have slept well but there was too much noise from a going away party for Jerome which was held on our roof, and lasted till about 4:00 am. I passed on the party, but got to hear the bass line (and practically feel it at times) from all the music that was played, though it was two floors above me! Last evening I got a call around 9:00 pm that a child had a high fever. The nurse, Salamawit, is an English speaker who I normally understand well in person, but other than the fact that the child had a fever I could not seem to get any more information out of her that I could understand. A bit frustrating, but I would have probably gone in in any case, and the child is okay. Needless to say I also have trouble understanding the French speaking staff over the phone. I am really enjoying the hospital work, even with these frustrations.

I am not sure how well I have described the "hospital." It consists of three large tents, some kind of heavy canvas with a waterproof surface, and one smaller tent. One tent is for the most serious cases when they arrive, an intensive care of a sort where we can have intravenous infusions, oxygen, and close monitoring with two nurses for at most 11 children. When the acute problem improves the kids pass to an intermediate tent for stabilization and to start growing, then finally on to a third tent to put on some more weight before heading home.

The small tent is a sort of overflow place when there are a lot of kids, like now. We have been generally close to our capacity of around 50 as there has been an outbreak of diarrheal disease, probably just a seasonal thing as we get into the fall season (95 degrees Fahrenheit!). The "doors" to the tents are flaps that people constantly enter and exit, and the tents have been full of houseflies. The mothers place light fabric loosely over their children when they sleep during the day, and use mosquito netting at night, but still a lot of time is spent brushing away flies.

One really sweet sight has been that of mothers taking their little toddlers, once they are recovering, to use tiny potties of various colors outside the tents. To see the little kids sitting on their little toilets, with their mothers in their brightly colored wraps, then the mothers washing their tiny bottoms, and often these are the same children who arrived practically unconscious two days earlier. Nice. I mentioned the one baby dying, I also was present a couple days ago when another died. Mother very stoic, had been expecting her child to die. They had arrived during the night when Dr. Alfonse was working, in very critical state. No tears from her at the time, but I have no doubt she mourned her loss. So I say this after describing the lovely sight of children getting better, it's a rough life for these little ones here but the vast majority are doing okay.

Why things have to be this bad in places like this is another question. I think about all the well babies I have seen over the years, how they came in for their check-ups during infancy, weight monitored carefully, immunizations 100%, with the most rare exception thriving. Thriving. That is what we expect in the west, and rightly so.

Anything less is "failure to thrive." Here the goal for many is to survive, and it is clear what failure to do that means.

The drive to the hospital during the day is relatively pleasant. We pass by a green area, where some trees grow, and there are some small streams. Kids are playing football (soccer) in the hot sun, apparently quite unfazed by the heat.

Last night I had a haircut at the local barber shop, right down the street from our house. It is run by Indian people. Brian had offered me the use of his trimmer, but like many people I enjoy the visit to the barber or hairdresser (interesting metaphor isn't it, dressing the hair?). So my reward for the visit was great. My head was buzzed, then once I convinced my barber that I wanted it shaved he started squirting various liquids on my head, shaving cream, and ultimately a nice shave with a straight razor (with disposable blade). Next a scalp massage. Next a massage of neck and shoulders. Finally he took out a tool that looked like a whisk that was open in the middle, allowing the metal wires to open out, and he ran this over my head a few times, causing a "shivers down the spine" experience. Wow. The price was about 4 dollars and 50 cents, and needless to say I gave him a tip! This will definitely be part of my routine here.

That is probably quite enough for now.

Hope you are all well! Dave

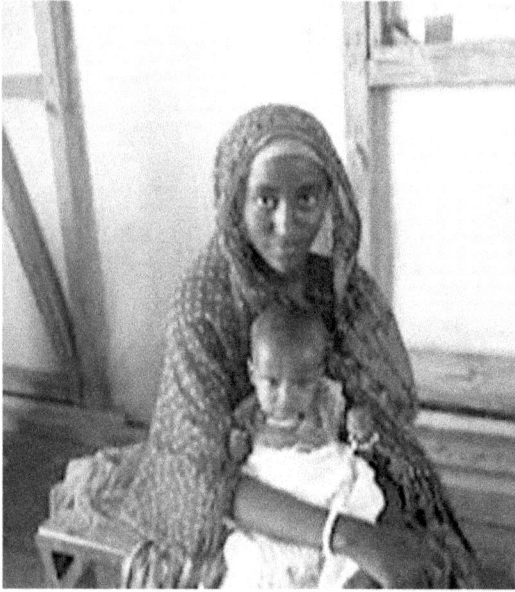

Lovely Mom and babe

Hello,

All continues to go pretty well here with a couple
of minor problems. I really was not sure I would have
much to write about this week. My weekend on call
went fine, it is actually good to have a routine that
includes working on the weekends. I also had been
looking forward to having this weekend off, and yes
it is good to be off. I have had a little cold for the past
several days, many here have had it. I was getting
over it when last night I was stricken by a bout of
diarrhea. I had been assuming that I would have less
of a problem with giardia here, less exposure to local
people trying to be sociable and serving lemonade
made with local water, as in Darfur, but no such luck.
Within an hour or so I was sure that it was giardia, so
I started treatment right away, and downed a liter of

oral hydration fluid. So now I feel much better!

Went for a walk this morning for the first time, very refreshing psychologically. Most of the crew here use the MSF car to travel even short distances. I like to walk, so this morning I got off to a good start by walking to my barber shop and having a repeat of my great haircut experience of last week. A 20 year old man from Yemen was there hanging out and he engaged me in a religious conversation. He observed that I have a beard, and wondered if it signified an affinity toward the muslim faith. He spoke French well, but there was still plenty of room for miscommunication, but to me it seemed the conversation went quite well, though I believe at the end he was trying to teach me Arabic so I could recite certain important phrases from the Koran. I rather enjoy having religious discussions here as in other places.

After a refreshing head shave and massage of scalp, neck, and back I walked to an Ethiopian restaurant I had been to a couple times. Dr. Emma's going away party was there, and people like the place. I had met the owner, an interesting Ethiopian character named Tedress, who has lived in Djibouti for 21 years. He is 59 years old and was previously in the Ethiopian military. He tells me there are 100,000 Ethiopians in Djibouti. I drank a great Ethiopian coffee with him around noon. He was already drinking whiskey, needless to say he is an Ethiopian Christian! He tells me that many Americans from the military base come to his place. I have seen many French people there. French soldiers have their families with them here, one often sees families with young children. After spending an hour with him I walked over to our office where I am at present.

The main refreshing quality of my walk involved being on the same level as the local commoners, who likely will never own a car of any sort, not to mention the big land rovers MSF is famous for. It also helped me to orient better to where we are in the city, as I had been to these places — barber shop and restaurant — only by car before. Saying hello to people, older folks and little kids, was nice.

The work this week has gone quite well. For the medical folks we had a case of miliary tuberculosis (TB) in a two or three year old. There is a referral center in town where we send kids who we believe may have TB for chest x-ray and consultation. The rate of TB is very high here. It is often hard to diagnose in children, they may not have a cough, and the only signs may be general failure to grow well, diarrhea, or unexplained fever. We have had a couple of kids so far who were not gaining after a few weeks of nutritional treatment, and have started improving after beginning treatment for TB. Generally the kids are doing well. Last weekend was the Muslim holiday of Eid, and all the mothers and children were dressed up. I took a lot of pictures for the first time here. Maybe I can figure out how to send along a few!

Tonight Nazet will be cooking a special meal, and the plan is to watch a movie on the roof after.

Someone has a device that can project DVD's. Sounds good to me. Hope all is well your way.

Siempre, David

Hi,

Rarely a dull moment here. The days fly by, I have been here over a month now. I am on call again this weekend. Last night I went with the crew I work with to a concert of Yemeni musicians, several singers, a keyboard/synthesizer player, and a really good guitarist. This was at the French Cultural Center of Djibouti, where the night before I had heard two American jazz musicians, a singer from Chicago named Keri Chryste who now lives in Paris, and a guitar player, Jeff, from Los Angeles and now Paris. The jazz was quite good, as was the Yemeni music. There were a lot of young Yemeni fans in the crowd who stood and clapped like young Americans at a concert. Quite fun to see. There were maybe 150 or so people there in all.

So I got home around 11:30 pm, happy that I had not been called. Fell asleep fast, woke up around 5:00 am hoping to go back to sleep for a couple hours, phone rings and one of the kids who had been doing well the day before had become extremely ill, so off I go, not even time for coffee! So I get there and the nurses have already started an i.v. which is great as the child really is just about dead, absolutely limp, cold hands and feet. So after a bunch of i.v. fluid and several antibiotics the child is sort of stable when I leave five hours later. I would have had to go in and see all the sicker children today anyway, so the five hours included seeing them. One child who yesterday had been in about the same shape as the child of this morning got worse again, so I was hopping back and forth between the two of them. My driver and friend Farad saved the morning for me by going down the street where an Ethiopian woman was selling coffee and getting me one "to go," which arrived in an old soda bottle. It was great Ethiopian style coffee! So I will go back in a couple of hours to check on things.

I have started really trying to get a smile or even a laugh out of the kids (not the ones who are struggling to stay alive of course, but after they have been in for a few days and start recovering). These malnourished kids do not smile a lot as a rule. I try common things like playing peek-a-boo, sticking out my tongue, dancing around, etc. The one effect that has been almost 100% is to get a laugh out of the mothers, who remarkably tend to smile a lot anyway. I remind you that these are women who have next to nothing of material value. When I am able to get a child to smile (and in only one case laugh) it is a great reward.

I read a document that Brian my Australian friend downloaded from the internet about the present state of the economy and government of Djibouti. It is not very pretty. The president is a despot who changed the constitution so he could have another term, rigged the last election, crushed opposition in general and specifically suppressed any protest during the Arab Spring era. He has made his daughter chief of staff (something like that couldn't happen in Maine, could it?), his mother is in charge of something, etc. Of course he is a great American ally in the War on Terror. There is something like 70% unemployment, 31% of the population is malnourished, not much good news in the report but I know from experience that a new gigantic supermarket named Casino (any ironies there?) just opened where you can buy practically everything that is available in Paris, from beauforte cheese to cognac. I tell all the guards and drivers that it is time for a French revolution style change of government here. They laugh, they all know what a crook their president is.

One of the chief imports to Djibouti is Khat, accounting for fully 10% of the country's imports. It is the leaf of a tree from Ethiopia that has a stimulant quality, and a mild narcotic property as well. After the daily shipment, it has to be fresh to work, by airmail in the early afternoon,one sees along the roadside many women with small tables with a blanket covering their wares, the fresh khat. I am told that a dose costs about six dollars. It appears that many adults, if they have the money, spend their siesta chewing on the leaves and relaxing. One of my drivers encouraged me to join him last weekend. I am going to pass. Apparently the stuff is legal here. We are not allowed to use the local taxis, as there are many accidents, as the drivers all take a break for the khat before returning to work for the late afternoon and evening. A literal example of "the opiate of the people"?

I watch the French soldiers walking with their families, women and children, riding bicycles, acting like normal people. The American soldiers stay on the base, and if they go out, travel in Hummers as if in Afghanistan or Iraq. An American I met who works at the embassy (not Chad from a previous report) told me that the US soldiers smuggled a prostitute onto the base wrapped in a rug, apparently keeping her there for some time. I hope they paid her well. The good news is that these soldiers were fired, as was their commanding officer, so occasionally there is a variety of justice in the world. Maybe it is for the best that the US soldiers remain on the base.

I am feeling very well, thank you, really enjoying the work, actually more than my other missions as it is really quite busy and essentially 95% clinical. There are a few regular meeting that are tedious, not at all useful, and last 2000% too long, but aside from that the job is very good. I have, as usual, become very friendly with many of the national staff—drivers, guards, cooks, cleaners, nurses, nutritional workers.

This has always been a great fringe benefit of the work for me in all of the places I have been.

Walking over here to the office this morning a door opened and out stepped the Djiboutian guard for the building, not MSF, just a random Djiboutian worker. After I said hello, I did a double take as I read his tee shirt—MSAD 46 in the middle of a heart, and some kind of message like "we care for our kids". For those of you not from Maine, this would be a shirt created in Maine for a local school district. Crazy coincidence, eh? So I spoke briefly with him about the connection. The shirt was clearly a give- away via some charitable route.

So the other day I am walking from one tent to another at the hospital and I see a tiny child standing alone, maybe 15 months old. So I squat down to his level and start "talking" with him. In a couple minutes he starts walking towards me and reaches out his arms to be picked up.

On that happy (and for me uplifting) note I end.

Siempre, David

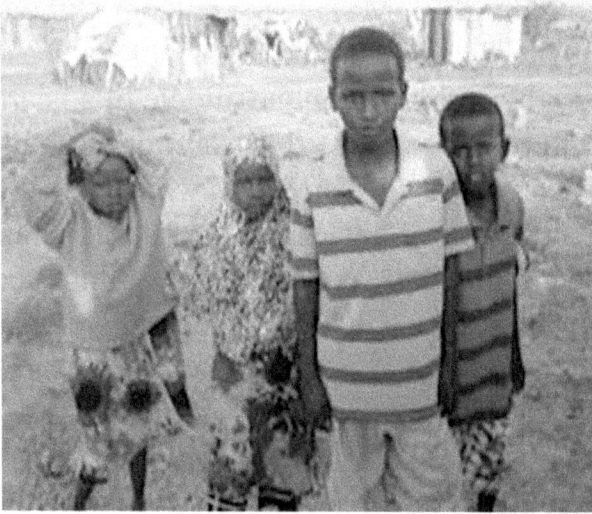
Beautiful children, wretched slum

Sent: November 25, 2011

Subject: Djibouti 6

Bonjour!

Happy Thanksgiving to all my US friends, always a little sad to miss my favorite holiday.

Interesting how these reports seem to write themselves. During the week I wonder if I will have anything much to say, and I make little notes about mundane things to include (and I always include them), but some thing or two seems to happen that provides a major point good for a few words.

The week was fairly uneventful as far as the babies go, generally doing well, none died, many went home. From time to time I see herds of goats traveling on their own. I noted this in the Congo, but it seemed more natural in such a rural setting. Here in a city of 500,000 they still roam untended. I always ask the drivers to explain how this works. Either the situation is so normal to them that they do not understand my question, or I do not understand their answer—in any case these goats seem to know where they belong at the end of the day, but I do not know how! Across the street from out house there is an open lot which is also an open dump of sorts, informally, full of plastic bottles and other trash. The goats like to visit there, as do several people looking for something of value to them. I saw the same man, relatively young, on 2 occasions pushing an old, rusty wheelbarrow and looking closely at objects in the dump. He was working pretty hard at it. He was not begging, but as I walked right by him on my way home I gave him a coin worth about 75 cents, and he seemed appreciative. I did not want to be insulting to him, and apparently I was not.

I started teaching an informal English class for any interested members of the MSF staff, first class was last Monday. Unfortunately there was a conflict with another meeting and only 1 person came. It was fun, will try a different day next week. I made a couple handouts and we spent time talking in English. Fun.

All the women at the hospital, except the Ethiopians, wear wraps and cover their heads, and some are veiled (eyes only) but no burkas. At first it was quite disconcerting to me to address veiled women, just not used to it and probably a bias that they may be extremely religious, but I am over it now. Very interesting experience seeing only the eyes, a lot of information conveyed by the eyes. Someone asked me about the nature of the material these women drape themselves with in such a hot climate. It is the lightest of cottons, as one would hope. I am sure I would be more comfortable if I were dressed like them, even with a veil!

Yesterday afternoon I was sent on a mission by my co-workers to find information about scuba diving here. After some travel and missteps the driver and I found the place. There will be no diving this weekend, as the boats were full, but maybe we will give it a go on my next weekend off in two weeks. As I was leaving the dive place I was approached by a women who looked to be a local, head scarfed in colorful wrap, until she spoke to me in perfect American English with no accent. It was clear from the start that she was upset. She apologized and said she approached me because I looked European and she saw me getting out of the MSF car. She was originally from Los Angeles, now living with her husband and 20 month old child in Germany, but at the moment I met her desperately stranded in Djibouti. She had flown there, leaving her child and husband in Kenya, to do some academic research on Somalian refugees. The contact person who she was supposed to meet was nowhere to be found, she had no place to stay, and her present goal was to get back to her family in Kenya.

She was happy to learn that I was from the US. She seemed truly shocked that I did not hesitate to give her the relatively small amount of money she needed to change her return flight and make a payment at the airport in Kenya. She told me that clearly God had sent me to her. I told her that I am a secular humanist. She still was appreciative, and invited me to visit her family in Germany, which I would like to do. The curious thing for me is that she would find it so remarkable that a fellow countryman the age of her father would want to help her with an amount of money that would equal about dinner for two with wine in the US (not at a fancy place!). I could not imagine not helping her.

This morning Nazet invited me and Beatrice to join her for breakfast. She said it would be a surprise and that I might not like it (she knows my politics). Turns out we went to a five star hotel called Kempinsky Palace, google it if you like, high security with gates and guards. Very lovely place on the ocean, flowers, nice swimming pools and beaches. Nice grand piano also which I played on a little. At first I was quite uncomfortable there, not my style under the best of conditions, but I could picture my tiny babies with their desperately poor mothers. I had an image of bringing them all there. Then I had a literary epiphany of sorts. I thought of Holden Caulfield in the last scene of Catcher in the Rye, where the title of the book is explained. Holden imagined what for him would be his perfect job. He would stand at the bottom of a cliff in a field of rye, with children playing at the edge of the cliff, and he would catch them when they fell. That is my job now, trying to catch these little babies as they are falling from this life.

It actually was relaxing to spend a couple hours there, if not wholly politically correct. I had a coffee. Most of the people there were French soldiers over from their base to swim in the pool for a small fee. One would have to be very wealthy to stay there, about 500 dollars a night I think. Nazet bought my coffee. There is a young couple from somewhere in South or Central America who sing there every night, Lisa sings and Rolly plays guitar. I met them and I may be joining them on the nice grand piano there. More later!!

The airport is close to the hospital, and too often I hear the harsh sound of military aircraft close overhead. I started visualizing how terrifying it must be to be attacked by planes spraying bullets and dropping bombs. This got me thinking about the US invasion of Iraq. I was sitting in a bar in New York City with Steve Quint when we saw the live coverage of the US attack on Baghdad. "Shock and Awe" it was named by the US military, like the most dark and ominous writings of George Orwell. We were both shocked by the whole affair I dare say, and to describe it as awful would be a grotesque understatement. And what was the headline once on Time magazine? Why do they hate us (US)?

To close on a more optimistic note, there is supposed to be a protest against the government here next Friday. It will be met with ugly police and military force in all likelihood, but this kind of heroism on the part of common people is inspiring, right up there with Occupy Wall Street (and it's many variations) for my money!

Be well and bon courage! David

Hello Out There!

Quite an eventful week. There was a very difficult day which I will describe, but some fun stuff first. I played a little jazz at the fancy place, Girl From Ipenema sung in lovely Portuguese. Sadly learned that the couple who perform there are leaving, to be replaced by some Eastern European band. May be all for the best. Last week I bought a footah (?spelling), the skirt that men wear here. It is very comfortable. I always wanted a kilt, but here the footah is much better. In any case, I wore it to my jazz debut and apparently it does not fit with the dress code for the bar where I was playing. My friends had to argue with the staff to let me stay. I was oblivious to all this. It made me more than a little cranky, the place is much too rich for my blood in any case, so good riddance.

The people I work with, national staff, are very appreciative of little things. Muriam, the women who cleans the office and makes coffee for everyone there, referred to me as "my brother" because I brought the dirty coffee cups down to her kitchen. People forget common courtesy when they have servants. My parents taught me better than that. Muriam also became my second English student, a bit of a greater challenge as she is illiterate, but speaks French very well. I made her an alphabet with pictures, like the youngest students use. It was not a work of art but was appreciated by her, needless to say.

Funny I haven't mentioned the traditional medicine that is practiced on the babies here. Most of them have white scars on their bellies and/or backs, some in relatively pretty patterns, others rough and ugly. They are all made by placing the burning end of a small piece of wood on the skin. Like torturing someone with a lighted cigarette.

I rather regularly now offer to the mothers my medical opinion on the practice.

This is my weekend on call. It is off to a good start, as I slept last night without interruption. I have seen the children already and all is relatively calm. Because it is the weekend I wore my footah in. The mothers and staff thought it was pretty great, only positive feedback, guess it affirms their culture a bit. I explained that it was the same in the US, on the weekend if a doctor has to work he might wear shorts and a tee shirt. I will be more professional tomorrow.

Two days ago two children died. The first one arrived dead, one of two little girls, sisters, who were brought in together. The second is doing okay but barely survived. They had a relatively brief illness with severe diarrhea, made us worry about cholera, but we are able to test for cholera and it was not, just an overwhelming diarrheal illness.

I first experienced the death of a child first hand in my residency over 25 years ago. In fact, until working in Africa, I had not seen a child die since. That child had an incurable congenital condition and was in the hospital in Rochester, New York for a kind of hospice care, as sadly the situation was too difficult for the parents to have the child at home. The baby was about six months old, and died in the hospital with the nurses and myself in attendance.

A couple of hours after the child arrived dead I was transferring a child to the more intensive area, as she had developed worsening diarrhea and needed intravenous fluids. As I was tending to this child, Beatrice called out that there was an emergency. Apparently a child who had been in the hospital for a couple days also had developed worsening diarrhea. The staff had been unable to find an intravenous site, and they were in the process of trying to insert a feeding tube to give fluids when the child stopped breathing. I had not been involved till this point. The child was clearly in bad shape, at first the pulse was okay but breathing was very shallow and ineffective. I started assisting the child's breath with mine. Beatrice found this bag and mask apparatus which was about five sizes too large and completely ineffective, so I continued the mouth-to-mouth, old fashioned approach. You want to picture that this is on a small single bed in our 11 bed ward, all the mothers are there, nurses are helping, Alfonse has arrived and eventually starts doing chest compressions as the child is clearly dying. The underlying problem was circulatory collapse from dehydration, so our efforts were probably in vain from the start. When we decided that the child had died, I asked someone where the mother was. She had been sitting silently beside me through the whole episode. I probably did the mouth-to-mouth for about 15 minutes all told. Can you imagine this, sitting and watching? So after there is the problem of trying to express something to the mother across cultures. It is practically forbidden for a strange man to touch a woman, and I am used to this by now, but what to do. I sat beside her for a bit, tried to gesture that I was sorry for her, then touched my head to her shoulder twice, just made it up on the spot.

So the next day I spoke with a very interesting man whose child was in the ward the day before. He speaks French fluently, unusual for the parents of our patients. I told him that it had been a hard day for me the day before, told him that it was often difficult to know what to do across cultures, and he told me that what I had done was appropriate and respectful, and that he had been impressed. Just lucky for me I would have to say.

I told Lois that other day that it is hard for me that there is not someone here I can confide in with difficult emotional situations like this. I really am getting to be good friends with Brian, but he is 25 years old and not yet a good candidate. Alfonse is an African doctor and it is all business. The flavor (literally) of my experience is as follows. There is not much in this life sweeter than a baby's breath. When I was doing the mouth-to-mouth thing it was a bizarre combination of experiences. The process, breathing into a baby's mouth, was not at all unpleasant, while the overall situation was horrible.

So after writing this, I will close with the observation that I am really loving the work, feel closer every day with the children and parents, and am getting to be very successful at eliciting smiles from the kids (and mothers). Toward the end of one day, maybe the one in question, I saw a mother sitting with her baby in the shade, no one else around. I sat down beside her and tried to be goofy with the baby, this time without much success, so I just sat for awhile. Very comfortable and comforting to me.

Hope you are all well. Have a great weekend!
Dave

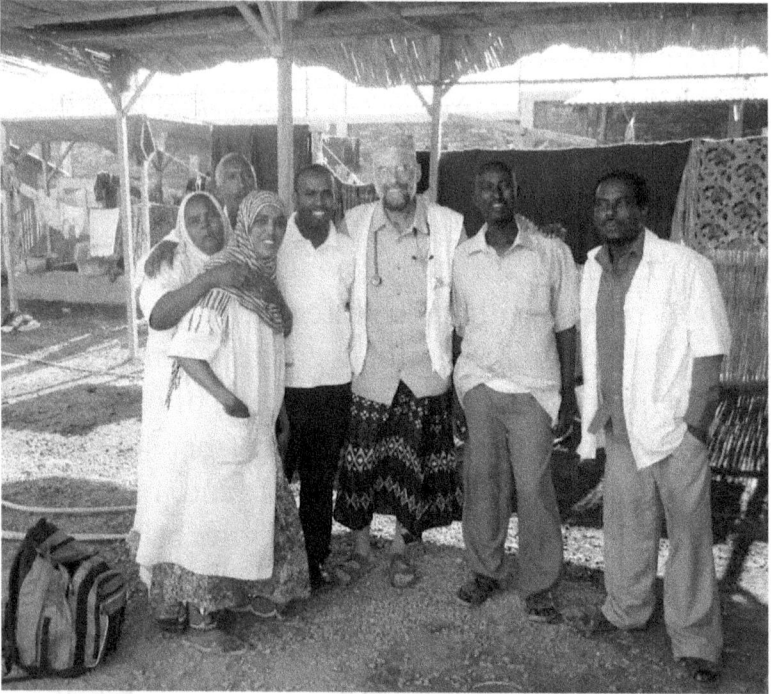

Team Djibouti!

Sent: December 9, 2011
Subject: Djibouti 8

Hello to Everyone!

It is very peaceful in the office today, only guards and drivers working. When I came in one of the drivers who I like and talk with a lot came with me into the medical office where I now sit. He sat patiently while I read emails, then started talking about some of his concerns with the MSF project shutting down. He clearly feels comfortable with me, most workers would not feel empowered to accompany an expat into their office, and frankly at first I felt a little uneasy because it is so uncommon, but I quickly came to my senses and behaved like a proper human being. I am not working this weekend. Funny how the work catches up with one, I seem to be getting enough sleep, started running some in the mornings before it heats up, just a half hour at a slow pace, but by the end of my 12 day stretch of work yesterday I was beat.

Fell asleep in the barber chair getting my weekly shave! And there has been a lot of evening socializing as the Head of Mission, Calil, will be leaving soon. He is the African from Mali, and will be replaced by Claire Peterson, a woman, and my guess is not an African, but who knows? I will find out soon enough. In the meantime there were going away parties two nights running, including last night, and one more this Sunday put on by our group. These are fun affairs which include mostly non-MSF people, mostly Africans working with other NGO's, wives and children (not being sexist with the wives thing, there are many African women working with the NGO's but none of them come with a spouse), and a few white guys from places like Scotland and Canada (one US, moi). So I guess I missed my usual 9:30pm bedtime a few nights. This morning I cooked omelets for the expats, went over pretty big. I may go to a beach close by this afternoon and do some swimming, and Brian and I are booked to go scuba diving tomorrow. Almost forgot, I am invited to a wedding tonight, the daughter of Nahda our house cleaner. Should be fun and very interesting, as they say.

When I work I am speaking either French or English with the nurses, and they in turn speak the native languages—Somalie, Afar, and occasionally Ethiopian—with the parents, so I spend a lot of time listening to the sounds of spoken language without comprehending the meaning. I have always enjoyed listening to foreign speech. We also spend a lot of evening time at a pool hall, Brian and I, playing 8-ball. This place has mainly Ethiopian workers, so I hear a lot of their language. The differences in sound are stark. The Somalie language is harsh, it always sounds like people are fighting but they generally are not. Reminds me a little bit of German, harsh and guttural. By great contrast is the Ethiopian language. When I hear it spoken in the female register it is birdsong, lilting and lovely. Curiously when these same Ethiopians speak English it sounds like they are frightened or upset, the lilting in English not fitting with the meaning of the words, upward inflections which suggest alarm to the English listener. How curious and interesting is that?

So I have learned most people's names after almost two months, and this has been no small challenge. There are still a few I do not know, guards I do not see often, logisticians who work mainly at the office. The problem is that most of the names are new to me, even after Sudan. The Congolese had mainly European names. So for your entertainment I will include a partial listing of my friends' names here, as taken from an official MSF document, so the spelling should be fairly accurate. Moutamar, Elme, Mako, Nahda, Youssouf, Fozia, Houssein, Fardoussa, Kaltoum, Madina, Ahmed, Souad, Omar (what a relief!), Ali, Nima, Fathya, Fouad, Madina, Rami, Kadija, Farhan, Moussa, Ikram, Mouhoubo (means love in Somalie), Mohamed (thank god), Fatouma,

Djama, Chihab, Ibrahim, Saada, Leila, Abdourahman, Moustapha, Abdour- azak,Oubah, Saredo, Mawlid, Hawa, Awa, Amina, Rouklya, Rachid, Abdoulkader, Zahra, Ismael, Faiza, Mariam, Hodan, Barkad, Ali-nour, Hibo, Aden, Souleiman. Get the idea?
But my favorite name is that of a lovely Ethiopian nurse who speaks English well (yes, always sounds distressed, I tried to express this idea to her and think she understood). I do not have the written name so the spelling may be off, but here goes. Salamaweet. Means "I am peace." How great is that?

So on that uplifting note I close. Be well and be peace, David

Sent: December 22, 2011
Subject: Djibouti 10 (Happy Birthday Arlen!)

Hello!

I am starting this on the 22nd, but will send it off
on my usual Friday schedule, which will be my son
Arlen's 30th birthday. I have been thinking about this
date for the past several weeks, as I do every year
(same thing when the 27th of September approaches,
Rob). Barely a moment goes by here that I am not
reminded of how similar people are from all over this
world. A couple days ago I was talking with Hussein,
one of the nutritional workers at the hospital. He is
23 years old and has a four month old son. We were
talking about the powerful experience of witnessing
the birth of a child. I was telling him that I can close
my eyes and vividly see the birth of both of my
children. We had no trouble sharing this common

195

experience, and many others.

Very difficult day today for me. I had hoped to tell a story with a happy ending but not to be. About a week ago the most malnourished child I have seen so far showed up, a girl, Hamda, three years and five months old, weighing 13 pounds (6 kilos). Nice weight for a four month old. The child had never seen a doctor or been in a nutrition program. This history made me think right away she must have a chronic condition, here likely tuberculosis. She became extremely ill soon after she got to us, was very dehydrated, and continued to have diarrhea. She was relatively stabilized with intravenous fluid, but when I returned in the afternoon she had taken a turn for the worse as no one had been able to find an intravenous site for many hours. She had become hypothermic (low body temperature), a sign of severe infection and/or dehydration to the point of circulatory collapse.

There is a procedure to use to get fluids into a child when one cannot find a vein. It involves placing a needle into the upper tibial bone (shin bone), and till last week I had only practiced this on a chicken bone. It actually is a lot easier than locating a vein in a dehydrated child. The child improved with the fluids, we ultimately found another vein or two, and Hamda was somewhat stable for a couple days. We sent her to the TB center and she was diagnosed with TB and treatment begun. Unfortunately her infection was far advance, including the pulmonary TB, and when the nurses called me this morning saying her breathing rate and heart rate were decreasing I was sure she was dying, and sadly I was correct. I got to the hospital around 5 am, saw the child, then sat with the mother, Fatuma, and my nurse friend Chihab, and discussed the situation. Fatuma of course had been there from the beginning, including knowing that I had placed a needle in her child's bone.

The father had also been around quite often, as had two other children in the family, both in good health, one younger and one older than Hamda. She understood well how grave the child's condition had been, and was not surprised to hear that Hamda was dying. She thanked me for trying to do everything we could for her child, and she kissed my hand. I had thought that I might lose it if this child died, but the courage of Fatuma gave me enough strength to keep things pretty much together. We went back into the tent, then the mother left, leaving the child alone. Hamda was unconscious at this point and breathing slowly. I sat with her holding her tiny, cool hand, feeling that she was somehow comforting me. I asked Chihab if the mother had left for some cultural reason, but no, she was just washing Hamda's clothes. She returned, as did the father, and they sat with Hamda as she died.

The routine when a baby dies is that the family is driven home in the MSF car. I made this trip this morning. The car drove deep into the slum where many of our patients live. I had never seen anything quite like it. "Homes" built out of rubbish, surrounded by rubbish. Children getting ready for school. We were soon surrounded by many children, interested in us. I took several pictures of them, which they enjoyed looking at. I also photographed some of the slum. I hope to be able to send off some of these pictures in the near future. While there we were approached by people asking us to transport a young woman to the hospital who they feared had appendicitis. We did this, of course, but our presence there was random, otherwise it would have been an hour's walk.

So I write this on a Thursday afternoon because we will be going off to the Isle of Mousha again tomorrow, leaving quite early. Thank goodness I do not have to work this weekend, really need the break. On Christmas Eve I will be making black pasta for the crew here, with Gorgonzola (or the closest blue cheese available) walnut salad and garlic bread. Someone is making a desert and someone appetizers and someone in charge of drinks. Should be fun, I look forward to the cooking. This will be a replay of the meal I made in Khartoum, and many times in the US. Thanks, Mary!!

Sorry to be sending a sad story for the holidays. All the other children are doing well, I get many smiles, bonjours, hellos, and nabats from the mothers and quite a good number of smiles from the children. I feel drained and exhausted today but invigorated and very much alive the bulk of the time. Loving the work here, cannot ask for much more than that.

Now it is Friday morning and I am getting ready to leave for a day of relaxation and scuba diving.

Had my weekly haircut early, great relaxation after the week. Hoping that you are all having a wonderful holiday season.

Siempre, David

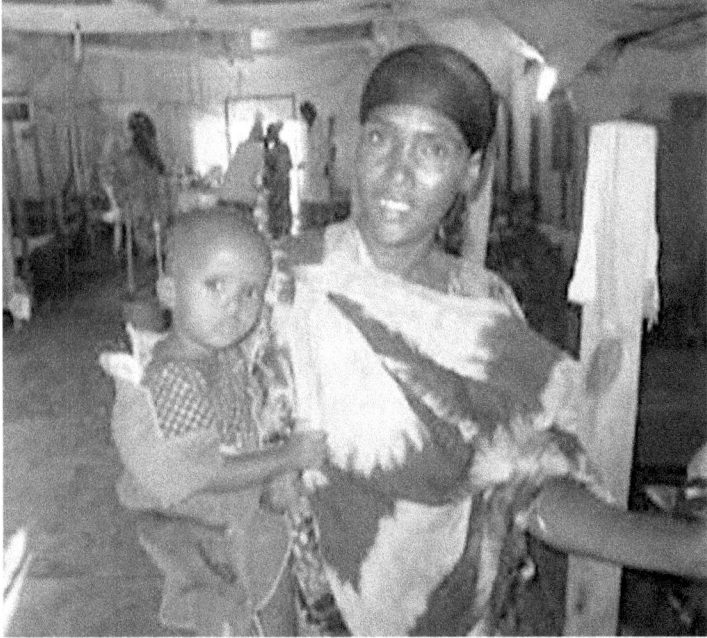

Two beauties

Sent: December 31, 2011
Subject: Djibouti 11

Hello!

No Internet in our office yesterday, so I am running late! We still do not have it, but I am visiting the office of a friend, Brian from Ireland, who lives in a place close to the President of Djibouti's house, so perhaps there is a stronger effort here to keep the local services up and running!

I have a lot of notes on things to write about, but as usual yesterday morning at work there were some most interesting events that I had planned to tell about, and I guess I will try today, though they are not as fresh in my mind. I am a bit tired today, in the midst of my final day of three consecutive of work.

I arrived as usual at the hospital yesterday,

wearing my footah as is my habit on the weekends when I am working. The nurses as usual were very friendly. I now know all their names, which continues to impress them. I also address the mothers and their babies by name, which I guess is unique. Their names are written on their charts, so it is no great effort on my part. So since it was Friday, our weekend, I was the only expat working, and I see only the sickest children and others with acute problems, which really does not take very long. So the nurses and nutritional workers invite me to have tea, one goes to their home nearby to make the tea, and they sit me down.

Foad, one of my nurse friends was raving about how much the mothers like me, in large part because of the name thing. I told him I think that using a person's name acknowledges that they exist and are important, and not using it sends the opposite message. Shortly after there was a discussion about religion. Moussa asked me about my religious beliefs. I had already talked to other nurses about beliefs, and they started saying something to him, I think reflecting accurately what I had said to them. I repeated that I believe in all religions as long as they are trying to do good in the world, I believe that all religions are essentially the same, and that the Golden Rule is probably all one needs to follow. I need a consult from my friend Alan, but I was listening to a program on religion a year or so ago and there is a famous story about a Jewish Rabbi who is asked to say in a few seconds what is the most important lesson (or some such, I know I am botching the details), and he repeats the Golden Rule. On this same program the fact was presented that the earliest know recorded statement of the Golden Rule come from China around 4000 years ago. I passed this news on to my friends here, along with the notion that if most people were subscribing to the rule we would not have these warplanes flying overhead or these children suffering, for that matter. Nice way to spend a weekend morning.

There is a very lively and interesting street life here. When I go running at 6:00 am in the morning the place is starting to wake up. I run past little tent-like structures that are peoples homes. The bread man comes by honking a little horn to attract business, some French soldiers run regularly as do a handful of Djiboutians. One morning I walked early to our office, a route I had taken 100 times later in the day. In the morning a place that I thought was a persons home in a vacant lot was actually a bustling "restaurant" with maybe 25 people eating food——probably omelets, doughnuts (made on the spot), and drinking tea. This morning I got to work at the usual 7 am, made a few visits, then stopped while the cleaning ladies did their jobs in the tents. I went to a similar "restaurant" just outside our hospital and had breakfast with a bunch of the staff.

We sat on large, empty powdered milk containers, which also served as tables for the dishes. The "building" is constructed of small round branches or small trees tied together to make a frame, which is covered by old rags, scraps of plastic. The food is cooked in an old wok-like pan, over charcoal, which is inside another trashed container, a little larger than the powdered milk cans. As I was sitting waiting for my omelet, watching a goat graze outside, I observed that there was not one single material thing in this restaurant that would not be in the garbage where I come from. It was very comfortable for me to be eating with my friends there. I gave an informal consult to a mother, not one of our patients, her child was quite grown up compared to ours, who wanted me to look at the x-ray that was taken of her child, and the list of medicines prescribed. All most interesting. The nutritional assistant who I had come to eat with bought an omelet for this anonymous child because she said she was hungry. Nice people here.

May have mentioned before that Brian, my co-worker from Australia, and I often play pool at a place close to us. I have become very friendly with the people who work there, Sisay from Ethiopia, Sali, a man who is a great cook from Yemen, Charko, a guy from Djibouti, Hawa and Zahra, two Djiboutian women, and Unkilo, the guard.

These people live a real-life sitcom, often laughing, occasionally fighting, working together. I play pool for free with them, smoke shisha (tobacco in a hookah for the uninitiated) with them on occasion, also for free, and generally relax and talk about life in general. It is a great mental break for me, going there. We also watch a lot of Hollywood movies dubbed into French.

Medical news. Think we are seeing some cases of

methicillin resistant staph pneumonia. Had a case that I thought was a great success, in the hospital for four weeks, two weeks of i.v. cloxacillin and gentamycin, then another week of oral cloxacillin, doing great with no fever for a week, lungs clear, went home and returned in three days as sick as initially. I restarted cloxacillin, gentamycin, and ceftriaxone, and the child did not improve one iota in 48 hours. Actually getting worse and I am getting depressed.

Had a brainstorm and added oral trimethaprim sulfamoxazole (works well for resistant skin infections), and child is without fever in 24 hours, plus clinically much better. We will see.

We will have a New Year's Eve party at our house tonight. There is a little security concern this weekend in particular in the downtown areas, as Djibouti just sent some soldiers to Somalia to fight against the Al Shabab forces there (militant Islamists), who have threatened to have some sort of revenge against Djibouti. No one expects anything to happen, but we will hang at home and invite some other NGO guys over. It will be a low key night for me, as I will still be on call, but may try to stay up to toast the New Year, as I have the day off tomorrow.

Well, quite enough for now. HAPPY NEW YEAR!!!!!!!!!!!!!!!!!!!!!!!!! (I will be celebrating 8 hours before the eastern US)

Siempre, David

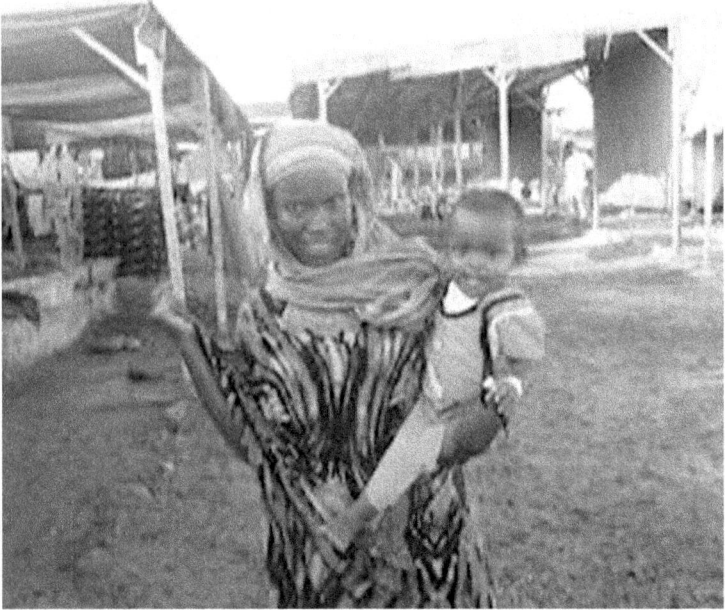

Mother and babe

Hello,

Writing early again this week, as will be off early tomorrow morning for another day of scuba diving. Hope you all received the pictures I sent. Some of the mails bounced back to me, apparently because of the attachments, but I later heard from others that they also did not get the pictures. I sent four separate emails, each with about 12 pictures. If you did not get them, try to get someone on the list to forward them on to you, as I have already asked a couple people to do for those I knew did not receive them.

Pretty good week of work here, all the children are doing quite well at the moment, though as usual there are a couple of hard cases that could go either way. On the positive side I discharged a child today who had been in the hospital for about five weeks, minus the three days she was home after the first three weeks. This is the case I mentioned where I believe she had a resistant staph pneumonia. Will never know for sure, but what is certain is that this seven month old was very close to dying twice in the past month, and was smiling and waving at me when she went home today.

I really like the way people carry themselves here, it is fun just to watch people walk, a very relaxed and easy gait, fairly effortless. As I write the effortless word I am reminded of two of the nurses, Said and Foad, who both had polio as children and who walk with some difficulty, but really relatively little. They both have awkward gaits with one very weakened leg, but they practically throw themselves around, keeping up with everyone else.

Many of the French soldiers and their families hang out in our local pool hall, as do other French people who live and work in Djibouti. I struck up a conversation with an older man named Gilles, probably early 60's. It was just a friendly conversation about nothing special, life in general, where we come from. A few days later as I was shopping in our local grocery store a voice spoke to me from behind and it was Gilles. Such a normal experience back home, running into someone you know while out shopping, but so uncommon here, it felt really good.

Not really a lot of news today. I feel pretty settled into a routine of work and recreation, the time flies by. New Year's Eve we had some other NGO friends over, Claire made a fondue which was good, we listened to music, I tried unsuccessfully to get people to dance. I truly like all of the Djiboutians and Ethiopians I have met here, some I consider true friends. This is identical to the experience I had in Darfur and the Congo. Also identical is the relative conflict with some of the westerners, on our team and others. Some people come to this work with a leftover colonial attitude which I find despicable at best. One woman who works with an NGO here I cannot stand. On our team I love Brian, Claire is fine but a little quirky, Alfonse is a goofy character, Nazet is a bit inscrutable and can be aggressive in a strange sort of way, and Beatrice has become a real problem in her relationships with Brian (he hasn't talked to her in about 2 weeks, except in meetings and to give her hell once), and Alfonse (she drives him crazy, he is happy to confide in me). I get along okay with her, but a couple days ago she was trying to do some teaching with one of the nurses and was contradicting something I had just told him (she was 100% wrong). I lost it a bit with her. I made peace with her a bit later in the day, but she is a real challenge, specializing in the passive-aggressive approach to life.

Well, on that somewhat unpleasant note I am looking forward to my weekly trip to the barber. There will be another soccer game on Saturday which has been hyped up a bit, a grudge re-match between the medical staff and the logistic staff, who won the last match 7-1. I am really looking forward to playing, will find out if my regular running will pay some dividends!

Hoping all is well your way.

Siempre, David

Sent: January 14, 2012
Subject: Djibouti 13, Friday the 13th

Hello,

I will begin by saying it is now Saturday the 14th.
I am working this weekend, and on the way to the
hospital yesterday I was telling Adenis, the driver,
about our (US) superstition about the day, and I guess
I made the mistake of saying that for me I felt the day
was not unlucky.

I wrote this message yesterday but it was lost in
the process of looking for contacts to send it to. This
was the least unpleasant of the unpleasant events of
the 13th. At least now I know the whole story of the
day, so here goes.

Last week a guy from France, Laurent, arrived
to present a program to the staff here on how to be an

effective supervisor. In general I have not had much of a good experience with such programs, but he seemed like a nice guy so I decided to put my bias aside and give it a try. Turns out the program was great, he is a fabulous teacher and lovely person, I got to have lunch twice with the national staff in restaurants of their choosing, places the expats never go (great to mix it up a bit), and I really learned a lot. The down side was the program went from 8:30 am till 5:00 pm, and I had to get to the hospital around 6:00 am daily for five days to try to get the work there done. This worked out okay, but by the end of the week, Thursday night here, I was beat, but it was my turn to be on call for the next three nights (tonight will be the last of these). I was smart enough to go to bed at 10:00 pm, had one minor call around 2am, and was sleeping soundly at 6:30 am when Friday the 13th began for me.

The call from the hospital told me a child who had been doing well, and was in the less ill part of the program, was suddenly in a coma. So I get ready, luckily there was some old coffee for me to slosh down, and I head in. When I arrive the nurses have done a great job, an i.v. is going, they have checked the child's sugar and it was low, he has received some sugar and is awake. So far so good. I review the child's chart and find he had a fever the day before, he is a tiny child of 9 pounds (4 kg), he had only been treated with oral medicines for his gastroenteritis, so I decide to treat him aggressively with intravenous antibiotics, and keep him in the intensive care area for the day at least. I finish the rounding (on Fridays we only visit the sickest kids and talk with the nurses about any problem cases, and see them). I finish up around 11:00am and head here (our office), after some fruit and yogurt, to write my email. After reading and responding to a few emails the internet takes a Friday the 13th break, so I decide to go into town and visit one of my Ethiopian friends, Mesei.

Within 10 minutes of my arrival the hospital calls saying there is a very grave case. Now sometimes the nurses overreact, but not on Friday 13. I head back to the hospital and find a good candidate for the sickest living child so far, a nine month old, Mohammed, unconscious and barely breathing, the history being incessant diarrhea for two days. No one can find a vein at first for the i.v., so I perform my second interosseous procedure (2 for 2), soon after the nurses get an i.v. going, fluids are started and antibiotics. Even with this the child is barely and at times not breathing, so for about 30 minutes I once again perform my mouth to mouth ventilator service. This works out better than the last time. I end up being continuously in attendance for 5 hours, till about 6:30pm. The child is fairly stable at this time, but certainly not well. As I am getting ready to go, I see a group clustering around another child. It turns out that the child from the morning has died, essentially without warning, as she had been eating fine during the day, had no fever, and all vitals sign were normal two hours before. Friday 13.

So I drag myself home and come to the office

to try again to write you all. This is the time, after completely finishing the email, I lose it equally completely while searching for a contact. More on this later.

Realizing that there are worse things in life than losing an email, I join Brian and Laurent for a great meal at an Ethiopian restaurant. Nothing went wrong there. On the drive home I decide to call the hospital to see how the new baby is doing. The nurses say they were just about to call me, he is not doing well. So another two hours are spent once again stabilizing the child, I get out around 11:30pm, and, after a shisha and a little piano playing, collapse into bed at 0015 on the 14th.

This morning I went for a run at 6 am, and got to the hospital at 7. On Saturdays whoever has the call does all the work, sees all the kids. I actually like this more than having the weekend off. It will be fun and necessary to have a break next weekend, fun to maybe go diving again, but my work here is more fun. This morning a child, Houda, who had been here for about four weeks, and who about 1 week ago appeared to be on route to dying, went home. Her mother was truly glowing, could not stop smiling. When she was ready to leave she made a sort of "victory lap" around the tent, saying goodbye to all of the other mothers, many of whom were also going home. This was unique in my experience, sort of a "high five" at having beat death this round. Very moving to me, I have a picture of her and her child and she insisted that one be taken of me holding Houda. Is it possible to attach a value to this? Two other children who looked to be dying a week ago now look to be recovering, so on balance the news is good. I love this work.

I have been thinking about moving to somewhere in Africa as a rather permanent (in the transcient nature of things) relocation. The people here seem to have a hard time not to smile. In three months I have seen less conflict among Djiboutians than I see in our house, among the expats, in a day. Will keep you posted. I certainly would want to spend a good amount of time in the US, but I am truly happy living here now.

To finish up with the 13th, Google in it's corporate wisdom has redone my email, so far resulting in the loss of my Djibouti Group and many individual addresses. Also lost was the automatic draft system, the loss of which led to my loss of the email yesterday. So I am asking you, Aileen, to look at the addresses on my last group mail and forward this mail on to anyone not on the present list. Thanks.

Hoping no one else had a Friday 13 similar to mine. Go Pats!!

Love, David

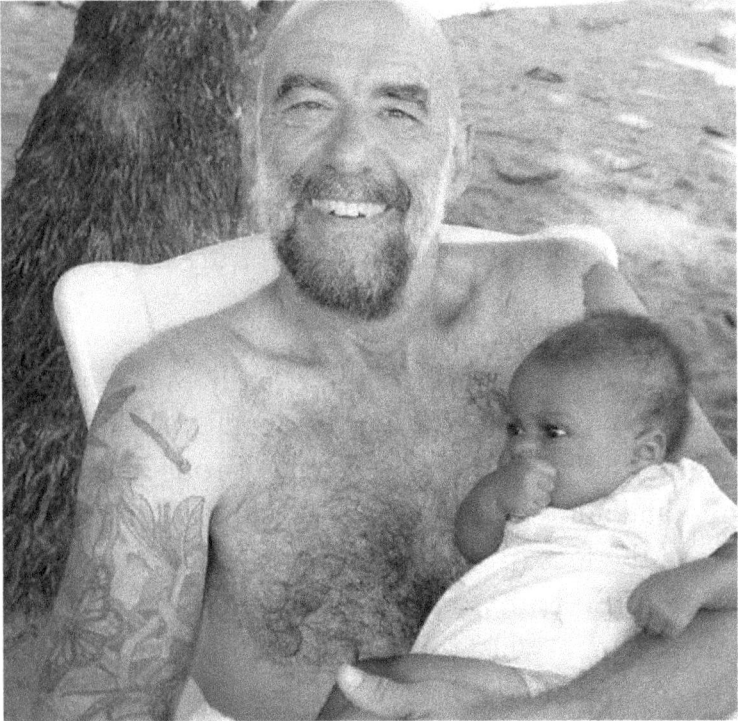

David and baby

Sent: January 22, 2012
Subject: Djibouti 14

Hello to all!

I once again had the annoying experience of writing a long email to you and having the internet crap out on me, losing it all. Not sure I have the energy to repeat it all but will do my best.

Not a bad week of work, but a bit over a week ago three babies died over a short period. Two of the deaths were probably unavoidable, but the third probably was. My doctor colleague Alphonse has a few problems, mainly he drinks too much, even when he is on call. Ironically he had not been drinking much when he was called for the baby I described last week, the one I had spent hours with, using both the interosseous infusion and the personal ventilator approach. The baby had been relatively stable and seemed to be going to live. The baby needed intravenous fluids again, and the nurses were unable to start an i.v. Alphonse arrived without a key that both of us carry (mine lives in my pocket, his should, too) so he was unable to use the interosseous equipment. Instead he tried to start an i.v. in the femoral vein (something the nurses I worked with in Congo were very good at, by the way), but he succeeded only in puncturing the artery on both sides. After a 30 minute round trip to get the interosseous materials, it was not long before the baby had died.

In the past I would have gone crazy after something like this, but the reality here is that the care that Alphonse provides is much better than that of the Djiboutian doctors. In this case maybe that doesn't seem like saying too much, but I have reached an acceptance of this reality, which certainly helps me sleep at night.

I was off this past weekend, and initially had planned to go scuba diving, but it turned out that the Djiboutians held a local election on Friday (our weekend), and it was felt that for security reasons we should stay close to home. The thought was that, like the surrounding countries, the Djiboutians might show some gumption and protest a bit. They did not, sadly. So I went to bed around 11:00 pm Thursday night, got up around 9:00 am and ate something, then went back to sleep until 2:00 pm. I was tired. This amount of sleep in a 24-hour period must be a personal record since I was one year old. I knew I was tired, but did not realize how much. The work goes on, it is compelling and rewarding, and one just keeps working, sleep is secondary. I like it!!

I was talking to a nurse friend, a man named Roble, a couple days ago. He is a mature and sophisticated nurse. He asked me about my children, and I in turn asked how many children he has. He answered, "eight, four living." The remarkable thing was the tone of his response, something like me saying "it is raining today." It took me a moment to regain my senses and tell him I was sorry. I am not sure he understood why I felt a need to say this. This brought me back to my experiences in Darfur, where all of the women had lost many children.

The difference is that in Sudan I was in the bush, and here we are in what would appear to be a modern city. The truth is that only the tiny percentage of rich people here receive decent health care. This for me is the greatest injustice in the modern world, and the problem the world should be working to solve. Some might argue for working to correct global warming, since there may not be much of a world left if this is not attended to, but for me a world where billions of people lack what millions see as their due is not worth saving, better let it return to the insects who will surely survive.

There seems to be so little will to do anything significant to help rectify this situation. The political

will is non-existent, witness the performance of
Obama, who campaigned on a bunch of politically
correct issues, then once elected has not raised
even his little finger against the corporate forces
that conspire to generate the ultra-wealthy and the
wretchedly poor. So ends my screed (as my mother
would say) for today.

Not much more to say, I am going to try to watch
the Patriots game on the computer, so wish me luck
(hope the Pats don't need luck today).

Siempre, David

Sent: January 28, 2012
Subject: Djibouti 15

Hello,

All goes pretty well over here. This is my
weekend of work, and it will morph into about eight
or nine days of solo work, as Alphonse will be on
vacation. Might be a little tired by the end, but as I
wrote, Alphonse's performance can be a bit shaky, so
in a way I am looking forward to being in charge for a
stretch of time.

These little kids are remarkable most of the
time. They show up weighting seven pounds at seven
months, you are afraid they will snap if you touch
them, you put a cup of milk in their mouths and they
guzzle it down and ask for more. They get better
and go home. Another group show up on the cusp of
death, infected in one way or another, and they either

die right off or they get a feeding tube stuck down their nose, struggle to survive for two to three days, either survive or not, then start a long, slow course of recovery, often with relapses, eventually drinking that milk from a cup and asking for more. We have a remarkable case, Hassan, who has been with us for about seven weeks. Today I transferred him out of the more intensive care area. For about the first month with us he did nothing but cry, practically continuously. Today I can get him to laugh.

A few of the mothers speak French, and it is a different experience getting a history directly without a translator. In all cases it is fun to sit with the mothers and discuss the care of their children. They are generally very smart and attentive to their kids, and often point out problems to me that are real. They also have a funny habit of drawing attention to what they think is a problem (like my child has a stomach ache) a day or two after this same child was practically dead form diarrhea and dehydration. Maybe a coping mechanism of some sort. My old friend Charlotte who I helped out when she was stranded in Djibouti is here to do some more research on the Somali refugees here. We are actually in the office together as I write. She is staying at our place for a couple nights, very nice to see her again.

Kenneth, the big chief from Geneva for our project, has been here this past week. Nice guy, originally from Ireland and/or Scotland (he says he is from both). Kind of bittersweet having him here as the project will be closing. All the staff continue to work along in relatively good spirits, knowing their days are numbered. A bunch of the nurses have asked me to write them letters of recommendation, which I have been happy to do with one exception. They hope to find work with another NGO.

I shaved my beard off a week or so ago, sick of trimming it all the time, just too hot. This gave the staff a chance to tell me how young I look now, and generally generated a bit of excitement. 100% of the male nurses approve, but surprisingly it's only about 50% of the female nurses. Maybe the 50% of female nurses who disapprove are the only honest ones?!?!

Soccer game this afternoon, I have to go soon and see the kids briefly before the game, there were a couple of very sick ones this morning but all was well when I left at 1:00 pm.

Hope all goes well where you are.

Siempre, David

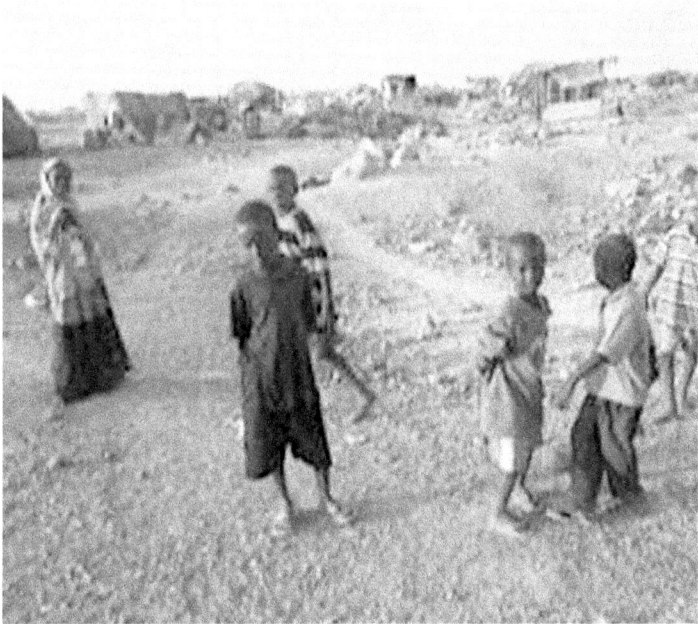

Beautiful children, wretched slum.

Hello,

I am now on the tail end of my hard week plus working solo. It really has not been too bad, but I will be very happy to have a week off starting Monday. All has gone really well with the kids. We have had a bit of a measles outbreak, my last experience with measles was when I had it as a child. Measles can be a real killer with malnourished kids, but ours are doing fine. We have three cases in a little isolation tent at the moment, and are vaccinating all the new arrivals at the moment.

The more medically significant development has been in the tuberculosis department. I had never treated a case in 25 plus years in the US, but now have been involved in the treatment of 20 or more

children. The treatment is very rewarding if started
in time. I think I talked about our frustrations with
the tuberculosis center we refer the children to.
They come back with x-rays that look like textbook
pictures of tuberculosis, but without treatment. Instead
the doctors order antibiotics against other possible
infections, and say come back in two weeks. One case
was so obvious that Dr. Alphonse went in with the
x—ray and discussed it with the doctor, who admitted
he must have missed the boat on the x-ray. So the
treatment was begun a week late and the child is
struggling to live at the moment. With Alphonse gone
I went in to talk with the TB doctor, Dr. Kamate, a
nice enough fellow. I convinced him to start treatment
on one child, but sadly this week too late start was
really too late, and the child died soon after. More
recently, I believe thanks to Kamate knowing my
face and knowing that I am looking at his work, he
has started treatment promptly on a couple of cases
which are now doing well. I should have gone in there
months ago, but my predecessor Dr. Emma had never
met this man, leaving any complaining or questioning
to Alphonse, so I stuck with that approach until now.
I will continue my more aggressive (but very tactful
I might add, not my usual fiery self) approach from
now on.

Today is the birthday of the Prophet Mohammed.
Not a giant holiday here, but on the local TV station
there was an interesting summary of the main
precepts of Islam as presented by Mohammed. One
could have substituted the teachings of Jesus for all
of them, of course the Muslims include Jesus as one

of their esteemed prophets, he is well represented in the Koran. This TV version also included several quotations very positive toward Christians, including them among the believers. Quite welcoming, I am not sure most Christians return the favor.

In a more obscure spiritual realm, as some of the pictures I sent attest, there is an overabundance of trash in Djibouti. I have asked a few of the nurses about this, and they acknowledge it as a cultural problem, people simply throw trash willy nilly everywhere, no matter how educated they might be. My Ethiopian friends are quite shocked by this, as apparently there is a different standard in Ethiopia. A lot of the trash consists of pastel colored plastic bags that blow all over in the wind. Many of the buildings here are surrounded by walls with barbed wire on top. As I was driving somewhere, looking out the window in a spaced out state, I saw many of these bags caught on the barbed wire, fluttering in the breeze, lovely pastel colors, and the effect was like a very long row of Tibetan prayer flags. Pretty Zen, eh? Preferable to get rid of the trash and barbed wire and raise a few proper flags, if you ask me.

So GO PATS. If they win Morrison buys me a gallon of top notch Massachusetts beer (he is so cocky he is giving me seven points).

Siempre, Dave

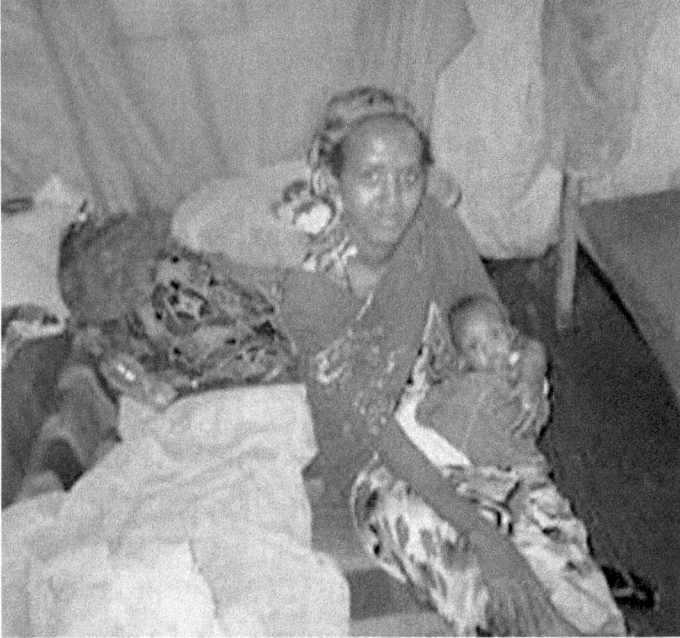

Two more beauties

Sent: February 12, 2012

Hello,

Briefly, I return from a great vacation to the news I will be leaving tomorrow. It is a long story I will not be telling by email. The good news is I will be seeing some of you sooner than expected.

Hope you are all well. I am fine, not to worry about me please. This means I have spent four months doing great work here (my assessment), and leave six weeks earlier than planned (my original contract was only till January 15, so one being an optimist would say I got an extension).

Love, David

Closing Thoughts

Life is precious and fragile. I spent a year working in Africa, bringing all of my family doctor skills to a very different world, far removed from the high tech US medicine of my practice in Maine. What did I learn? How has this experience changed my view of the world?

Life is precious and fragile. I sat with dying people, most of them young children. I experienced the strength of parents as they lost children. I experienced the generosity of common people, sharing their meager material goods, but more importantly, sharing their boundless good spirit.

MSF fills a special niche in the world of humanitarian work. Historically all of their work was relatively short term, responding to medical emergencies resulting from natural or manmade disasters. Dropping in and out of people's lives for relatively brief but intense periods is both rewarding and frustrating. As a doctor in Maine I attended births and tended growing children, met older adults and helped them age and die. My African work lacked the continuity over years. More frustrating was the short-term nature of the programs themselves. Ironically, the only program I worked in that was intended to be long-term, the hospital in Darfur, ended when we were thrown out by the government of Sudan. The other two projects, in the DRC and Djibouti, were closed down as planned shortly after I left. Judging from the emails I received from colleagues who were at these projects when they closed, I was lucky to miss the painful process of packing up and leaving for good. There is a debate within MSF as to whether or not the organization should be involved in more long-term projects. Time will tell, but there is so much medical need in our world, both acute and chronic, that all efforts to help are good.

Personally, I am planning to settle somewhere in the world where I will be able to provide medical care to people who lack it. I am retiring from work in the US, a gradual process which began with my first international work in the Dominican Republic in 2002. One of my main goals as a citizen of the US was to "deploy" somewhere in the world in a non-military fashion. Having achieved this goal, life goes on. I look forward to the next chapter.

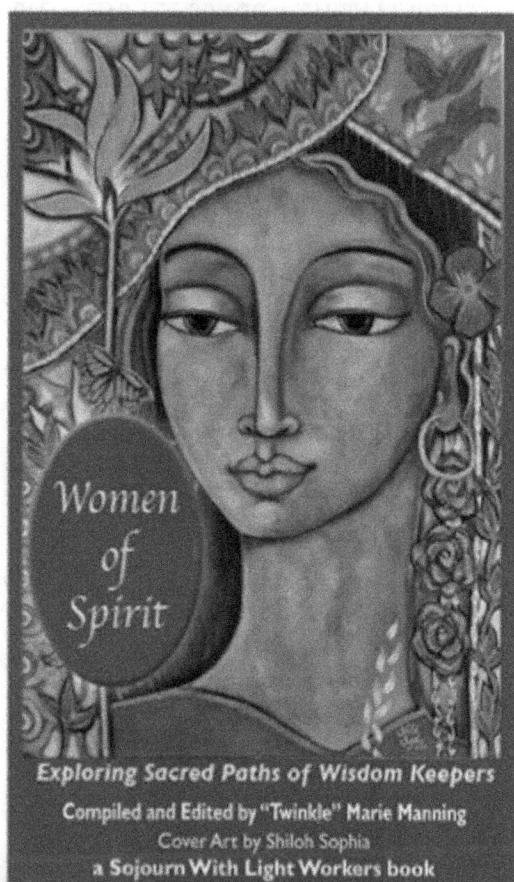

Women
of
Spirit

Exploring Sacred Paths of Wisdom Keepers

Compiled and Edited by "Twinkle" Marie Manning

Cover Art by Shiloh Sophia

a Sojourn With Light Workers book

This book is a compilation of women sojourners, sages, mystics, witches, shaman, medicine women, ministers, philosophers, therapists, life coaches, yogis, and more. Their journeys. Their stories. Their teachings and practices. Essays, Poetry, Art, Rituals and Prayers. This anthology is full of useful tools and powerful messages for everyone who is on a spiritual journey to embrace and enjoy. Originally published in 2014, this beautiful anthology has been recently revised and re-released. Beloved Contributors include:

• *Anna Huckabee Tull* • *Bernadette Rombough* • *Deb Elbaum*
• *Deborah Diamond* • *Debra Wilson Guttas* • *Grace Ventura*
• *Janeen Barnett* • *JoAnne Bassett* • *Judy Ann Foster*
• *Julie Matheson* • *Kate Early* • *Kate Kavanagh* • *Katherine Glass*
• *Kris Oster* • *Lea M. Hill* • *Meghan Gilroy* • *Morwen Two Feathers*
• *Rustie MacDonald* • *Shamanaca* • *Sharon Hinckley* • *Shawna Allard*
• *Shiloh Sophia* • *Susan Feathers* • *Tiffany Cano* • *Tory Londergan*
• *"Twinkle" Marie Manning* • *Tziporah Kingsbury* • *Valerie Sorrentino*

OTHER MATRIKA PRESS SELECTIONS

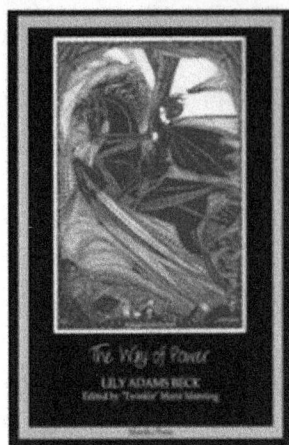

Seventh Principle Studies:
The 7th UU Principle is: *"Respect for the interdependent web of all existence of which we are a part."* Evidence to support such a principle is found within the pages of *The Way of Power.*

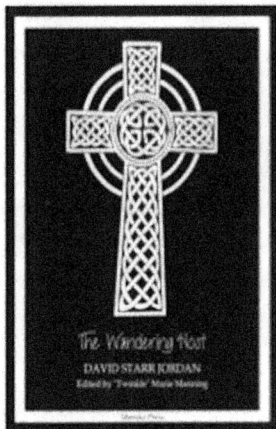

Sixth Source Explorations:
This allegorical story by David Starr Jordan is a tale about the search for spiritual meaning. Symbolic of Jesus Christ's ministry, it succinctly embodies the Unitarian Universalist Christian heritage and the fourth of the six sources we draw our faith from, namely that which calls us to respond to God's love by loving our neighbors as ourselves.

www.MatrikaPress.com

F

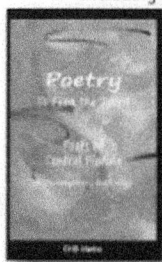

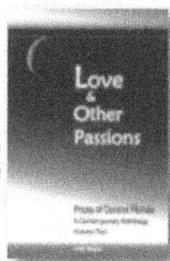

Coming Soon

Where the Sky has No Stars

A poetry anthology by Wesley Burton

Wesley's contemplative and imaginative poetry entices readers to face moments of transition. His words explore the inner depths of the psyche, the healing power of nature, and the soul's resilience to move forward out of darkness.

http://MatrikaPress.com/wesley-burton/

RECOMMENDED SELECTIONS FROM SKINNER HOUSE

Finding the Voice Inside: *Writing As a Spiritual Quest for Women*

Gail Collins-Ranadive offers forty practical and imaginative writing exercises that invite women to explore their uniquely feminine spirituality. Through writing of symbols, metaphors and truths of their own lives, women re-awaken to higher truths of their sacredness.

Reaching for the Sun

Rev. Angela Herrera's book of meditations, prayers and invocations provide inspiration to readers and serve as a resource to those seeking powerful liturgical words, grounded in the experiences of everyday life.

Evening Tide

This book of mediations by Elizabeth Tarbox helps readers to face the darker moments of life, the challenging circumstances that call us to live more fully even when we feel our most empty.

http://www.uua.org/publications/skinnerhouse

RECOMMENDED SELECTIONS FROM BEACON PRESS

Claiming the Spirit Within

This wonderful book, edited by Rev. Marilyn Sewell, is a beautiful sourcebook of poetry and prose. A rich and diverse anthology dedicated to the praise of life, it presents the sacredness that emerges when women immerse fully in living lives of spirit while embracing the physical. Its contents include more than 300 poems celebrating all aspects of women's lives. Contributors include Margaret Atwood, Rita Dove, Louise Erdrich, Tess Gallagher, Nikki Giovanni, Joy Harjo, and Maxine Hong Kingston.

A Chosen Faith: *An Introduction to Unitarian Universalism*

Authored by Forrest Church and John A. Buehrens, this book offers a an informative look at Unitarian Universalism. The authors explore the history and sources of this living tradition. For those contemplating religious choices, Unitarian Universalism offers an appealing alternative to religious denominations that stress theological creeds over individual conviction and belief. It allows room for individual interpretations of the sacred and encourages affirming diversity, personal choice, shared experiences, rites of passage, religious education and work for social justice.
http://www.beacon.org/

www.ingramcontent.com/pod-product-compliance
Lightning Source LLC
Chambersburg PA
CBHW051717020426
42333CB00014B/1027